REVIEW OF
INTENSIVE
CORONARY CARE

FIFTH EDITION

REVIEW OF
INTENSIVE
CORONARY CARE

FIFTH EDITION

Jacquelyn Deal, RN

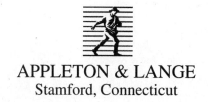

APPLETON & LANGE
Stamford, Connecticut

Copyright © 1996 by Appleton & Lange
A Simon & Schuster Company
Copyright © 1983 by Robert J. Brady Co.

96 97 98 99 00 / 10 9 8 7 6 5 4 3 2 1

Prentice Hall International (UK) Limited, *London*
Prentice Hall of Australia Pty. Limited, *Sydney*
Prentice Hall of Canada, Inc., *Toronto*
Prentice Hall Hispanoamericana, S.A., *Mexico*
Prentice Hall of India Private Limited, *New Delhi*
Prentice Hall of Japan, Inc., *Tokyo*
Simon & Schuster Asia Pte. Ltd., *Singapore*
Editora Prentice Hall do Brasil Ltda., *Rio de Janeiro*
Prentice Hall, *Englewood Cliffs, New Jersey*

Editor-in-Chief: Sally J. Barhydt
Production Services: Rainbow Graphics, Inc.
Cover Designer: Mary Skudlarek

ISBN 0-8385-8416-0

90000

9 780838 4163

PRINTED IN THE UNITED STATES OF AMERICA

Contents

Preface

Nurses—
closed shades—
hushed voices—
flashing lights—
buzzing alarms—

Come on in to CCU: *Scary.*
Now here's a closer view:
pleading eyes—
reaching hands—
healing hearts—
needing you—
Patients.

You are obviously interested in coronary care nursing or you would not be reading this. I hope to make this subject more exciting and more comfortable for you by taking you figuratively by the hand through the coronary care unit as you care for patients. You have the "Yellow Manual" (Dracup's *Intensive Coronary Care*) as your basic guide, but I hope this *Review* and workbook will help you organize your knowledge and increase your retention of all you need to know to function expertly in coronary care nursing.

Through the pages of this *Review of Intensive Coronary Care* I will share some of my ideas with you, ask you some questions to see if you understand the material, and try in a variety of informal ways to make your introduction to coronary care a pleasant and valuable experience.

I will assume that you work in, or will work in, a CCU and that you can observe what you are learning to make that learning come alive.

Since we can't actually sit side by side during this CCU course, our common meeting ground will be the 5th edition of *Intensive Coronary Care*. After all, any book that has sold thousands of copies and been translated into several languages must have something special going for it. By going through the book together as we review, we will be able to find out where you need more information and more review. This book is designed to help you sort out the facts, apply what you learn, and test your own knowledge. Here are a few of the methods I have used in trying to make this a useful guide:

Situations: Role-plays, dialogues, and case studies are presented. These are designed to make you feel "you are there" and encourage you to exercise your judgment and knowledge. Use your imagination to project yourself into these situations: make mistakes on "my" patients; then do it right on your own. At times, I will ask you to pretend that you are in charge of a CCU.

Questions and Fill-in-the-Blanks: In these pages you will find hundreds of specific questions to test your knowledge. In many instances they follow a programmed approach leading you step by step to a conclusion. Answers are provided so that you may check yourself. In the sections where the answers are shown in the right-hand column directly across from the questions, put a 2-inch-wide strip of paper over the answer column. Read the first question, answer it in your own mind, and fill in the answer blank. Then move the strip of paper down to expose the answer. Were you right? Congratulations! Were you wrong? Well, now you know what the correct answer is. Go ahead and complete the rest of the questions in this manner.

Application: You will also be invited to ask yourself and your colleagues questions, and then draw your own conclusions. Some questions are purely reflective; answer them in the context of your own situation and environment.

Electrocardiographic Rhythm Strips: I have selected a series of rhythm strips taken in my own coronary unit for us to go over together. I will tell you a little about the patients, and we will see what you would do under the circumstances.

Before we begin, I would like you to reassure yourself that you are not a complete stranger in foreign territory. Ask yourself the following questions, and as you think about your answers, realize how much you already know about coronary care nursing.

1. Have I seen or cared for patients with heart attacks?
2. Can I remember how those patients felt and acted?
3. Can I remember some of the problems they had?
4. Has a family member or friend ever had angina or a heart attack?
5. Can I list some of their symptoms?
6. What else do I know about coronary heart disease?

You are not really entering an unknown world. You have already had some experience in dealing with coronary disease. In fact, you probably know a great deal about this illness. We are ready to start organizing that knowledge and building on it. You, the learner, are unique. Use your own knowledge and skills, and let's build on those.

Jacquelyn Deal

REVIEW OF
INTENSIVE
CORONARY CARE

FIFTH EDITION

1

The Coronary Care Unit

THE PHILOSOPHY OF INTENSIVE CORONARY CARE *(pp. 1–3)*

Welcome to Intensive Coronary Care: a dynamic system, an evolving philosophy. On page 2, the author of *Intensive Coronary Care: A Manual for Nurses* (from now on called *The Manual*) says, ". . . individual coronary care units may lurch between the old hierarchical model and the newer collaborative model. . . ."

So, where are *you* starting from? Remember in the Preface I said we were assuming that you worked in (or had access to) a CCU and we would go from there. (If you didn't read the Preface, go back and do it now please!)

Review 1

In the old hierarchical system, to put it bluntly:

Hospitals and doctors bossed the nurses
Nurses bossed the ancillary staff (sometimes)
And everybody bossed the patient

Some three decades ago, Dr. Meltzer and others changed that with a radical step: they delegated responsibility to the nursing staff. Thus we find:

1. The nurse was expected to carefully _____ the patient and _____ monitor patterns.   *observe   interpret*

2. The nurse must be capable of making _____ about a course of action.   *decisions*

3. The nurse would have the _____ to carry out therapeutic actions.   *authority*

This is the basis we all start from. In Figure 1.2 of *The Manual,* we see the "new system" is based on:

4. _____ respect, _____ authority, _____ governance.   *Mutual   shared   shared*

5. In essence, it is a _____ model.   *collaborative*

(You may use any words meaning the same thing. Just grasp the importance of the concept.)

DESIGN OF THE CORONARY CARE UNIT *(pp. 3–5)*

Review 2

In pages 3 to 5 of *The Manual* you will find nine criteria for an effective CCU to help minimize "ICU psychosis" for the patient.

1. QUIET. Have you any idea how noisy a CCU can seem to the patient? In the "old days" of open ward unit, a patient would complain because we whispered at the desk at night. (And I do mean whispered!) When you become more familiar with your unit, you will tend to become noisier. Watch it!

2. VISUAL OBSERVATIONS for the nurse and PRIVACY for the patient. Not impossible, it just means to remember to shut the door and pull the curtains when your patient deserves privacy.

3 and 4. Patients are not only uncomfortable, they lose track of time, date, and place when criteria 3 and 4 are overlooked. You are the one who can change this.

5, 6, and 7. It's dream time! You may have to make do with less, but if you are in the planning or redesign stage, speak up!

8. Scream and holler in the design stage—electrical hazards are real. And the first time a patient says, "Hey, that bit me!" (ie, electrical shock), scream all the way to the top administration.

9. Check out your alarms. Imagine you are at the bedside and there is a sudden cardiac arrest. Can you get help without leaving the bedside? (Hollering your head off doesn't count!)

EQUIPMENT FOR A CORONARY CARE UNIT *(p. 5)*

Cardiac monitoring and ECGs, rest assured, will be covered in much more detail later on. For those who need it, I will invite you to a little review of coronary anatomy and 12-lead ECG.

EQUIPMENT FOR ASSESSMENT *(pp. 5–6)*

The Manual lists the equipment you should find in your unit. If you are unfamiliar with the equipment and procedures, get copies of the manufacturer's material and try to see the devices in operation. On page 5 *The Manual* refers to a low ejection fraction, which you will learn more about in Chapter 7. For now, ejection fraction equals the amount of blood pumped from the left ventricle compared to the total amount in the ventricle before it contracted. In heart failure the amount is less than 40 percent.

Review 3

1. Hemodynamic monitoring assesses the patient's ＿＿＿＿＿＿ and ＿＿＿＿＿＿ to treatment.

   condition   response

2. You do this by measuring pressure directly in the ＿＿＿＿ and ＿＿＿＿＿.

   heart   arteries

3. Equipment you should find in a CCU for hemodynamic monitoring includes:
   <u>special catheters and tubing</u>
   ＿＿＿＿＿＿
   ＿＿＿＿＿＿

   manometers
   transducers

4. In larger or teaching hospitals you may find two noninvasive measurements of cardiac output:
   a. ＿＿＿＿ ＿＿＿＿＿
   b. ＿＿＿＿＿ ＿＿＿＿＿ ＿＿＿＿＿

   Doppler ultrasound
   transthoracic electrical
   　bioimpedance

Assessment of Arterial Oxygen Concentration *(pp. 5–6)*
Review 4

1. You are asked to collect blood samples from Mr. Kardiak's femoral artery or other arterial lines. You would use a _____ collection tube to prevent clotting.

2. You would send the specimen to the lab in a container of _____ _____.

3. The specimen would be used to analyze _____ blood gases.

4. This is used to assess _____ oxygen consumption and metabolism.

5. This is important in assessing the patient for circulatory _____ and in following his response to _____.

6. Noninvasive measuring of arterial oxygen saturation can be done with a _____ _____ placed on an extremity.

7. It is most accurate when placed on a _____.

8. An invasive measure of oxygen saturation ($S\bar{v}o_2$) of mixed _____ blood requires a _____ _____ catheter.

heparinized

crushed ice

arterial

tissue

failure
treatment

pulse oximeter

finger

venous
pulmonary artery

EQUIPMENT FOR TREATMENT AND RESUSCITATION *(pp. 6–9)*

Defibrillator/Cardioverter *(pp. 6–7)*

We had better clarify some terms: we are talking about one machine with two uses.

A. An emergency life-saving measure (defibrillation)

B. A therapeutic measure (cardioversion)

Read the section on pages 6 and 7 in *The Manual* and then answer the following questions.

Review 5

1. One form of electric shock is called defibrillation. (True/False)

2. Defibrillation is used to terminate _____ _____.

3. Defibrillation is an emergency life-saving measure. (True/False)

4. Defibrillation is a term also used for elective treatment of arrhythmias. (True/False)

5. The second form of precordial shock is called _____.

6. Cardioversion can be used to terminate _____ as well as ventricular arrhythmias.

7. Cardioversion is an elective, therapeutic measure. (True/False)

8. The basic electrical principles of cardioversion and defibrillation (are/are not) the same.

9. However, _____ must be used at a particular time in the cardiac cycle.

10. _____ is not synchronized with any part of the cardiac cycle.

11. Both types of shock can be delivered by the same machine. (True/False)

True

ventricular fibrillation

True

False

cardioversion

atrial

True

are

cardioversion

Defibrillation

True

Pacemakers *(p. 7)*
Review 6

Pacemakers are covered in much more detail in Chapter 15, so for now simply check out the pacemaker equipment in your CCU.

1. You should find two general types of pacemakers:
   external: _____
   internal: _____

transcutaneous
transvenous

Take a better look at the transvenous pacing equipment in your CCU. Transvenous pacing is a two-way street.

2. The electrode(s) passed through a vein contacts the inner heart wall and transmits electrical stimulus (to/from) the heart.

3. The electronic circuitry senses electrical activity coming _____ the heart.

4. The power source or _____ can then deliver the pacing stimulus at just the right time.

to

from

generator

Respiratory Equipment *(pp. 7–8)*
Review 7

1. Mechanical respirators should be kept in the _____, not in the respiratory therapy department.

2. What kind of respirator do you find in your CCU? _____

3. Do you know how to use it? If you don't, get help from someone who does.

4. List emergency trays and supplies used for respiratory assistance that you find in your CCU. _____

5. Two older and very basic life-saving devices also needed are _____ _____ and _____ _____.

CCU

Ambu bags
suction equipment

Crash Cart *(p. 8 and Table 1–1)*
Review 8

You can use Table 1–1 on page 8 in *The Manual* in two beneficial ways:

1. Check your cart supplies against the list.

2. Check the medications you need to learn more about. We will cover drugs in more detail later, but why not get started now?

THE STAFF OF THE CORONARY CARE UNIT *(pp. 9–11)*

Review 9

If you are blessed with the role of staffing a CCU or providing education for CCU nurses, you will be especially pleased with the 5th revision of *The Manual*. If after reading this section, you feel inadequate, remember, we all did before we completed CCU courses. And many of us have enough humility (or honesty) to still feel inadequate.

This section does not need questions and answers, but let's discuss a few things from our viewpoint as nurses. A few of you may have the dubious/delightful/delirious privilege of helping set up a new CCU. Here are some scenarios.

1. Here comes the hospital administrator, Mr. Stuffer. He says, "You need one specially prepared RN for every 2 patients? Haven't got them. I will put two untrained RNs in. That won't do? Okay, one trained RN for 6 beds and I will find you 2 LPNs. You had better accept that; after all, it's more staff than any other place in the hospital." And off he stomps. His CCU is stuffed, not staffed! Your new CCU has special equipment; it needs specially educated nurses to run it.

2. How do you select the nurses for this special education? Ms. Purr Swaytion, the Director of Nurses, is selecting her staff: "Imogene, we will send you to the two-week CCU course so you can be in charge. Now, now . . . after all we have done for you, this is the very least you can do for us. And Gertrude, you will be in charge of nights. Imogene will teach you; we can't afford to send you both. My dear, you won't

refuse, not if you remember your annual raise. (Coercion seldom creates skilled CCU nurses.)

3. There are five aspects of nursing practice listed on page 10 in *The Manual;* CCU nurses are expected to _____, _____, _____, _____, and _____.

assess plan implement
evaluate communicate

PREPARATION OF THE CORONARY CARE UNIT NURSE *(pp. 11–13)*

Review 10

Now let's get practical. It is time to evaluate where you are and where you want to be as a CCU nurse. Consider the topics on page 12 in *The Manual.* What is your present level of knowledge? What level do you need as a CCU nurse? Then review the skills checklist in Table 1–2 on page 13 of *The Manual.* Which skills do you need to practice or review?

If you are in a CCU class (or reading this book alone), do you need extra help to reach your goals? If so, start getting it now. Find a clinical nurse specialist, a clinical educator, a physician, or other health professionals and establish mentor relationships. Get going! You CAN do it!

Coronary Care Nursing

ANATOMY REVIEW

Before we begin Chapter 2 in *The Manual,* let's do a brief review of the anatomy of the heart. Refamiliarizing yourself with some of the terms will help you sail through the next chapter.

Review 1

1. Fill in the correct names of the chambers, valves, and vessels as numbered in Figure 2.1. Cover the answers at the right.

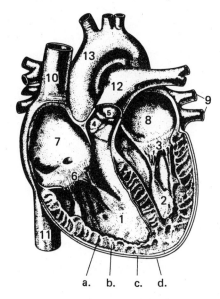

Figure 2.1. Cross section of the heart.

1. _____ right ventricle

2. _____ left ventricle

3. _____ bicuspid, or mitral, valve

4. _____ semilunar aortic valve

5. _____ semilunar pulmonary valve

6. _____ tricuspid valve

7. _____ right atria

8. _____ left atria

9. _____ pulmonary vein

10. _____ superior vena cava

11. _____ inferior vena cava

12. _____ pulmonary arteries

13. _____ aorta

2. Describe how blood circulates through the heart and major vessels. Use the appropriate numbers from Figure 2.1 for each part you list.

Venous blood returns to the heart through the _____ and the _____. It then passes through _____, _____, _____, _____, and _____ to reach the lungs. From the lungs it moves through the _____, _____, _____, _____, _____, and _____ to the body.

10   11
7   6   1   5   12
9   8   3   2   4   13

3. Name the three layers of the heart wall as lettered in Figure 2.1.

a. _____

b. _____

c. _____

endocardium
myocardium
epicardium

4. What is the membrane surrounding the heart? _____

pericardium

How did you do? If you are dissatisfied, why not dig out your old anatomy and physiology book and refresh your memory. When you are satisfied with your knowledge, go on to the next section.

Review 2

There are some terms you will meet briefly in this chapter that are fully explained in later chapters. If you aren't familiar with them and it bothers you, then you can turn to these pages in *The Manual* for more information:

ischemia—p. 55 (bottom)   necrosis—p. 58 (top, col. 2)
ventricular fibrillation—p. 213 ventricular standstill—p. 244
defibrillation—p. 216   stroke volume—p. 95
preload—p. 95   afterload—p. 95
ejection fraction—p. 95   myocardial contractility—p. 95

NURSING RESPONSIBILITIES IN THE CORONARY CARE UNIT *(p. 15)*

Review 3

"I am a Coronary Care Nurse." What will it mean when you can say that? It means hours of study and lots of hard, devoted work. It means hearing the patient's family say, "We feel safe with you here." And after an emergency, when the patient says, "Hey, I'm still alive!," it means indescribable ecstasy. As we find out more about your role in Chapter 2, remember, you, the beginner, are unique. Use your own knowledge and skills, and let's build on those. That is a quote from the *Preface* of this book. You are the best judge of your own current level of expertise. By now you should have a fairly good idea of where you are headed. So what are the *goals* of coronary care?

1. _____

preserve life

2. _____

prevent complications

3. _____

restore patient to maximum
    functional capacity

CONTINUOUS ASSESSMENT OF THE PATIENT'S CLINICAL STATUS *(pp. 15–18)*

Direct Observation of the Patient *(pp. 15–18)*

Review 4

Because the heart is the pumping machine for the body, you are very concerned with the problems an impaired pump might cause your patient.

1. Thus, you are going to observe your patient closely for any signs of _____ _____.

circulatory compromise

2. Areas you will specifically check are: _____, _____, _____, _____ _____, _____ _____ _____ _____.

skin extremities pulses
    blood pressure   heart and
    lung sounds

3. Your assessment will help you, first, to establish a _____ and then to identify any _____. Sounds like an old nursing adage you are probably familiar with: if you can recognize "normal," you can identify abnormal.

baseline
changes

Some of the baseline observations can be done while you are admitting the patient.

Review 5

Let's try admitting a patient. Dr. Hart calls and says, "I am sending a patient over from the office. I think he might be an MI, but he is not in severe pain right now. Admit him and then call me."

Answer these questions, and then read the discussion that follows.

1. The very first thing you will do when the patient arrives is _____
_____
_____
_____
_____
_____
_____
_____
_____.

ATTACH THE MONITOR. No 5-minute welcoming speech; don't demonstrate the call bell system; don't present the complimentary admission kit; don't even take his TPR—get the monitor on. Know your equipment so well that you can think about the patient's feelings and not the hardware connections.

2. While you are doing this you should _____
_____
_____
_____
_____
_____
_____
_____.

EXPLAIN WHAT THE EQUIPMENT IS ALL ABOUT. But don't expect him to remember; his anxiety level at this point is too high for that. During the rest of his stay in CCU, encourage him to ask questions and repeat explanations as often as necessary.

3. He may develop an arrhythmia at any time, so take an _____
_____
_____
_____
_____
_____.

ADMISSION MONITOR STRIP—stat! Later on when the doctor says, "Was he having these PVCs on admission?" you can show him exactly what the initial cardiac rhythm was.

4. What should you write on this admission monitor slip? _____
_____
_____
_____
_____.

WRITE THE PATIENT'S NAME, THE DATE, AND THE TIME ON THE STRIP. Many nurses also write the doctor's name on it.

5. While you are admitting him, what else should you be doing? _____
_____
_____
_____
_____
_____
_____
_____
_____.

OBSERVE THE PATIENT AND GATHER CLINICAL INFORMATION. If you know your equipment, you can attach it automatically and spend your time talking with the patient. Determine 1. type and degree of pain, 2. location of pain, 3. symptoms of heart failure or shock, and 4. general appearance and condition.

6. He may need emergency cardiac drugs, so it is a good idea to _____
_____
_____
_____
_____

START AN IV AS SOON AS THE MONITOR IS ON. If you have a helper, then do both procedures at once. Although you may be able to identify an arrhythmia and know how to

_____
_____
_____
_____.

7. When would you call the doctor? _____
_____
_____
_____
_____
_____
_____
_____
_____.

8. The doctor orders a 12-lead ECG. Why? _____
_____
_____
_____
_____
_____.

treat it, you are still lost without an IV for emergency drug treatment. Get this lifeline in place in a hurry.

AFTER YOU ATTACH THE MONITOR, HAVE THE IV IN PLACE, TAKE THE VITAL SIGNS, AND ASSESS THE PATIENT'S CONDITION. (In other words, WHEN YOU HAVE COMPLETED numbers 1 through 6 above.) Then you have worthwhile information to give the doctor.

TO DIAGNOSE AN MI. The monitor only tells you about arrhythmias.

Review 6

You have just settled your first patient when the ambulance team calls. "We are bringing in a bad one, don't know if he will make it." What do you do? Panic and get it over with. Then prepare for anything.

1. In preparing for the patient, you would put at the bedside the _____
_____
_____
_____
_____.

CRASH CART (including the defibrillator). Screen it if you feel it looks too frightening, but have the defibrillator plugged in and ready to go.

2. When the patient arrives, the first thing you will do is _____
_____
_____
_____
_____
_____
_____.

GET THE MONITOR ELECTRODES ON. If the house doctor wants to examine the patient and Respiratory Therapy wants to work with him, fine—but you shove in there and get the monitor working.

3. How about undressing the patient first? _____
_____
_____
_____
_____
_____
_____.

NO, INDEED! I saw a 42-year-old man go into cardiac arrest while we were undressing him. I am convinced that shoes and pants don't count. All you need is a bare chest with electrodes on, and you are set to save a life.

4. While you are putting the monitor on should you explain to the patient what you are doing and why? Even if he is in critical condition? _____
_____
_____
_____
_____.

YES, maybe he can hear you even if he is too weak to talk.

5. Why rush to start an IV? _____
_____
_____
_____
_____
_____.

EMERGENCY DRUGS MAY BE NEEDED—undoubtedly *will* be needed. And the IV line will be instantly available.

Skin (pp. 15–16)

Review 7

Now let's build on the knowledge you demonstrated in the last exercise and go into more detail.

A. Mr. Paul Paller is being admitted. You immediately notice he looks like a ghost.

1. Pale skin tone (pallor) can simply be caused by _____ or _____ temperature.

   anxiety   cold

2. If that is the cause, his skin color will _____ as your good nursing care makes him more relaxed.

   improve

3. Rather than just waiting, you examine his eyes: the _____ for pallor.

   conjunctiva

4. While you are admitting him, you examine the _____ of his hands.

   creases

5. Pallor (that is not due to anxiety or cold) reflects _____ oxyhemoglobin.

   decreased

6. This could be caused by _____, _____, low _____ _____, or infective _____.

   anemia   hypovolemia
   cardiac output   endocarditis

B. Cyndi Cyano is admitted and you immediately notice her bluish color.

1. Cyndi's nail beds and lips are blue. This is _____ cyanosis.

   peripheral

2. Of course, if it is 10 degrees below zero outside, that could be the cause. But you must suspect _____ cardiac output.

   low

3. You will want to further inspect Cyndi's _____ and _____ _____.

   tongue   mucous membranes

4. Blueness there is called _____ cyanosis.

   central

5. You will want to know if Cyndi suffers from _____ _____ _____, _____, or _____ _____.

   congestive heart disease   COPD
   pulmonary hypertension

6. If central cyanosis develops suddenly in a recovering MI patient, the cause may be _____ _____ _____ or _____ _____.

   ventricular septal rupture
   pulmonary embolus

7. You will also note skin turgor; this means the _____ status and _____ of the skin.

   fluid
   elasticity

8. When you touch your patient's skin, you hope it will feel _____ and _____.

   warm   dry

9. Cold, clammy skin is the hallmark of _____ _____. (And once you touch it you will never forget it.)

   cardiogenic shock

10. Cold, clammy skin can also result from pain and _____ cardiac output of _____ or _____.

    decreased
    angina   MI

Extremities (p. 16)

Edema

Review 8

1. Edema may be one of the first signs of _____ _____ _____.

   congestive heart failure

2. Look for edema in patients on bedrest in the _____ area.

   sacral

3. In patients not on bedrest, you note edema first in the _____ _____.

   lower extremities

4. To check edema, you press gently on the edematous area for _____ seconds.

5. A 2-mm indentation = _____+
   a 4-mm indentation = _____+

5
1
2

Clubbing
Review 9

1. Clubbing, related to cardiac conditions, is caused by _____ _____ _____ _____.

2. It could also be caused by _____ _____ _____.

3. Thus, it is a symptom of _____ rather than an acute condition.

4. Other signs of clubbing are _____ _____, _____ _____ _____, _____ _____, _____ _____ _____.

low arterial
oxygen saturation

congenital heart disease

chronic

bulbous fingertips   thick,
   hard nails   spongy nailbed
   straightened nail angle

Petechiae
Review 10

1. You might find petechiae on the _____ or _____, or under the _____.

2. You might (rarely) find Osler's nodes, which are nodes of the pads on the _____ and _____. (They are seen in about one fourth of endocarditis patients, so give yourself extra points if you find them!)

ankles   wrists   nails

fingers   toes

Complication of Inactivity
Review 11

1. If Mr. Kardiak remains on bedrest for a couple of days, watch him carefully for signs of _____.

2. You find these in the _____ _____, _____, and _____ _____.

3. Mr. Kardiak is at greater risk because of his _____ cardiac output.

4. Signs of thrombosis are _____, _____, or _____.

5. The real danger is that a thrombus could circulate and become a _____ _____.

thrombosis

lower extremities   thighs
   pelvic area

low

inflammation   pain   swelling

pulmonary embolus

Pulses (p. 16)
Review 12

Of course you know how to take radial pulses and a few others, but do you know where all seven pairs of pulses are located?

1. You palpate the pulses to assess _____, _____, _____, and _____.

2. Amplitude is rated on a scale of _____.

3. An absent pulse is rated as ___; normal pulse rates _____; and bounding pulses rate ____.

4. A bounding pulse is also called _____.

5. Mr. Kardiak does NOT have a pulmonary artery catheter but you can still assess the _____ and _____ in the right side of the heart.

6. You can _____ the _____ pulse; palpation might _____ the pulse.

7. You would inspect the neck veins with Mr. Kardiak at a _____° to _____° angle.

See page 16 in *The Manual*

rate   rhythm   amplitude
   contour

0 to 4+

0   2+   4+

hyperkinetic

volume   pressure

inspect   jugular   obliterate

30   45

8. Look for the venous pulse about _____ to _____ cm above the sternal angle.

1 3

9. If you find the venous pulse higher than 3 cm, it is a sign of _____ volume and pressure in the _____ _____.

increased
right atrium

10. This may be due to right _____ failure, _____ regurgitation, or _____ hypertension.

ventricular tricuspid
pulmonary

Blood Pressure (p. 16)

Review 13

1. You already know that blood pressure is determined by _____ _____ and _____ of the arterial walls.

cardiac output
elasticity

2. High blood pressure (hypertension) means a _____ BP above 90 mm Hg.

diastolic

3. Low BP (_____), is a persistent BP of less than _____ mm Hg.

hypotension 95/60

4. Which is more often a problem in CCU? _____

hypotension

5. If Mr. Kardiak has hypotension, you would carefully watch his monitor for _____, also known as _____.

arrhythmias dysrhythmias

6. These can decrease his _____ _____ and _____.

cardiac output BP

7. Severe continuous hypotension may be a warning sign that Mr. Kardiak is going into _____ _____ or _____ shock. (Two things you will learn to dread.)

ventricular failure cardiogenic

8. Treatment of hypotension is directed towards:
   a. normalizing cardiac _____
   b. giving _____ fluids
   c. treating low _____ _____

rhythm
volume-expanding
cardiac output

9. Two devices that you will learn much more about are the _____ _____ pump, and _____ _____ device.

intraaortic
balloon ventricular assist

10. Drugs that might be used for hypotension include inotropes. A drug with a positive inotropic effect is one which (increases/decreases) muscular contraction.

increases

Examination of the Heart and Lungs (pp. 16–18)

Review 14

1. The usual examination of heart and lungs involves the four methods of _____, _____, _____, and _____.

inspection palpation
percussion auscultation

2. You as a CCU nurse focus on evaluating any _____ in the patient's condition. These could indicate a response to _____ or be a _____ of the disease.

changes
therapy worsening

3. The lungs are auscultated to identify _____, _____, or _____.

rhonchi wheezes rales

4. If you are sharp, you can recognize these findings about _____ hours before they show on x-ray.

24

5. Thus, you can identify the beginning stages of _____ _____.

pulmonary congestion

6. You would use the _____ of the stethoscope and ask the patient to _____. Then have the patient breathe in and out slowly while you begin auscultation at the lung ___ ___.

diaphragm cough

bases

7. The heart is auscultated to identify abnormal _____.

sounds

8. Most important are _____ and _____ heart sounds, _____ friction rub, and _____.

3rd 4th pericardial
murmurs

13

9. You would use the _____ of the stethoscope starting at the _____ of the heart for 3rd and 4th sounds.

bell   apex

10. These are _____, _____-pitched sounds caused by vibration of _____ walls when blood rushes _____ the ventricles.

soft   low
ventricular   into

11. When the ventricles lose their compliance and dilate, _____ is heard during early diastole as the _____ valves open and rapid filling of the already distended _____ occurs.

S_3
atrioventricular
ventricles

12. In late diastole, the atria _____ and force more blood into the already distended _____.

contract
ventricles

13. This makes the (S_1 / S_2 / S_3 / S_4) sound. _____

S_4

14. The compliance of the _____ may be impaired after an acute _____ or in chronic _____.

ventricles   MI
hypertension

15. The sudden appearance of either S_3 or S_4 may be a sign of new myocardial _____ or _____ _____.

ischemia   heart failure

16. A rough, scratchy sound that increases with inspiration is heard if the patient develops a _____ _____ _____.

pericardial friction rub

17. It is caused by the pericardial layers (_____ and _____) rubbing together due to inflammation (ie, _____).

parietal   visceral
pericarditis

18. Listen for it at the _____ border in the _____ and _____ intercostal spaces.

sternal   3rd   4th

19. Table 2–1 (p. 17 in *The Manual*) summarizes heart murmurs. Your concern is not so much with identifying pre-existing murmurs as with _____ in those murmurs.

changes

20. If as Mr. Kardiak is recovering, you discover a new high-pitched, blowing murmur at the apex, you might fear the rupture of the _____ _____ of the _____ valve.

papillary muscles   mitral

You will find a diagram of the heart sounds (Fig. 7.1) and more information in Chapter 7, Review 13.

Electrocardiographic Monitoring *(p. 18)*

You will learn plenty more on this subject in later chapters. So for now, go shake hands with a monitor and while you're at it check into the "standing clinical protocols" in your CCU (most often referred to as *THE* protocol).

Hemodynamic Monitoring *(p. 18)*
Review 15

1. Poor Mr. Kardiak looks pretty puny this AM. Wouldn't you love to know *exactly* what is going on with him? There are two pressures you would like to monitor: cardiac _____ and _____.

venous   arterial

2. Hemodynamic monitoring starts with simple _____, something every CNA is taught.

BP

3. More complicated, invasive techniques measure _____ _____ _____ and cardiac _____.

pulmonary artery
pressure   output

4. To do this, a _____ is passed, usually through the _____ _____ or _____ vein to the _____ side of the heart.

catheter   internal jugular
subclavian   right

5. This will probably be done with the aid of _____.

fluoroscopy

6. The pulmonary artery catheters you will use for this will probably have _____ or _____ lumens (_____).

2
3   openings

7. Let's just get the basics of what you can do with this catheter now; in Chapter 3 you will learn more. One lumen allows you to measure pressure in the _____ _____; you can also inject fluid into this to measure _____ _____.

right atrium
cardiac output

8. You can use a second lumen to measure the pressure in the _____ _____.   pulmonary artery

9. You can _____ a balloon in the catheter and this lumen lets you measure pressure in the _____ _____.   inflate
left ventricle

10. Don't get lost! You are now able to measure three pressures: _____ _____, _____ _____, and _____ _____.   right atrium   pulmonary artery
left ventricle

11. With a thermistor, using a technique called _____, you can measure cardiac _____.   thermodilution
output

12. The third lumen is used to administer _____ or IV _____.   drugs   fluids

13. You may find your pulmonary artery catheters are a special fiberoptic kind that allows you to continuously measure mixed _____ _____ saturation.   venous oxygen

14. This reflects Mr. Kardiak's overall _____ utilization.   oxygen

15. Some catheters also have a _____ wire for temporary pacing. (Now if they would only teach that catheter to clean up after the doctors!)   pacemaker

16. You will use the hemodynamic monitoring information to _____ _____ and make other treatment decisions.   titrate drugs

17. You would expect to see Mr. Kardiak on hemodynamic monitoring if he develops any of the following serious complications: _____ _____, _____ _____, _____ _____ _____, or _____ _____.   heart failure   cardiogenic
shock   ventricular septal defect
pericardial tamponade

ANTICIPATION AND PREVENTION OF COMPLICATIONS (pp. 18–21)

Decreased Cardiac Output Related to Arrhythmias or Mechanical Factors (pp. 18–19)
Review 16

1. A basic goal of CCU is to prevent the two lethal arrhythmias _____ _____ or _____ _____.   ventricular fibrillation
ventricular standstill

2. Standing protocols authorize nurses to treat warning arrhythmias with IV _____ or _____.   lidocaine
adenosine

3. In addition to arrhythmias, nurses must be able to identify _____ defects on the monitor.   conduction

4. The treatment for this might be inserting a _____ _____ _____.   temporary transvenous
pacemaker

5. You must watch these pacemakers for failure due to _____ failure or _____ wires.   battery
disconnected

6. The second most frequent cause of decreased cardiac output are things that affect _____ _____.   stroke volume

7. Factors affecting stroke volume are _____, _____, and _____ _____. (More on this later.)   preload   afterload
myocardial contractility

Impaired Gas Exchange/Ineffective Airway Clearance (p. 19)
Review 17

1. When you admit Mr. Kardiak _____ blood is drawn and oxygen tension (_____) is measured to determine if he should be on oxygen.   arterial PaO_2

2. If he is _____ or has ischemic chest pain he probably would receive _____ to _____ L/m of oxygen.   hypoxemic
2   4

3. We have talked about many ways of assessing a patient's ventilation and perfusion. List as many as you can. _____

_____
_____
_____
_____
_____
_____.

See paragraph 3, p. 19 in *The Manual*

4. If oxygen by mask or cannula isn't adequate, be prepared to help with _____ and _____ ventilation.

intubation
mechanical

Fluid-Volume Excess or Deficit *(p. 19)*

Review 18

1. When the patient's cardiac output drops, the body increases its output of _____ and _____ hormone.

aldosterone   antidiuretic

2. This is meant to increase cardiac output by increasing _____ _____.

intravascular
   volume

3. However, this can result in too much _____ excess and cause _____ _____.

fluid   pulmonary edema

4. It is extremely important for you to keep accurate _____ and to be sure _____ is restricted in the diet.

I & O   sodium

5. Signs of increased fluid volume include:

_____

_____

_____

_____

_____

See column 2, p. 19 in *The Manual*

6. Increased fluid volume can be treated with _____ and _____ _____.

diuretics   fluid
   restriction

7. Be wary of giving too much _____ _____ in order to administer IV drugs.

IV fluid

8. _____ (too low blood volume) can result from excessive _____ or fluid _____.

Hypovolemia   diuretics
restriction

9. Signs of hypovolemia are: (List 4)

_____

_____

_____

_____

thirst

poor skin turgor

high urine specific gravity

hypotension

Sleep-Pattern Disturbance *(pp. 19–20)*

Review 19

There are 2 statistics cited from a study in *The Manual* that are real shockers. And as nurses we are too often part of the problem and not part of the solution.

1. In this study, NO patient completed a "natural _____-minute sleep cycle."

90

2. Sleep disturbances occurred every __ minutes. What can you do to keep this from happening in your unit? _____

_____

_____

_____

_____

20
See pp. 19–20 in *The Manual*

EMOTIONAL SUPPORT OF THE PATIENT

The Manual has excellent information on emotional responses and emotional support. Read it carefully. As nurses, we see these reactions in every one of our patients, and we should know them well. The following poem will help us to take a closer look.

Faces of Fear

How do we know the faces of fear that we see in our own CCU?
The mouths, do they open and close on the words
I'm afraid!
Will you help me?
I'm scared!
Not very often . . .
Not me, not to me
Strong, robust, roving, roaming.
To have to be fed,
Tethered down in this bed.
I'm a puppet with strings to my heart.
Ashen wife, tears held back.
They lie, those tests,
It's someone else.
Really, just somethin' I et.
Why me, why to me?
I'm a father with children,
Wife, life, love, longing . . . leaving?
Yes me, yes to me but . . .
Perhaps to stop smoking,
Be kind, gentle, loving?
Give my eyes or my kidneys . . .
Are they taking livers these days?
How 'bout it, God . . .
Two more years?
It's a deal?
What do we do with these faces of fear that we meet in our own CCU?
Our mouths, do they open and close on the words
You're afraid,
Can I help you?
I care.
Well, they should . . .
Fear all alone is so AWFUL—
Together: perhaps, not as bad?

—*Mary Bayer*

Together now, let's consider the emotional reactions we see in our patients.

Faces of Anxiety

Mr. Mild Anxiety: He is one of the rarest patients we see in a CCU. He has reached the stage where he has accepted his condition and has begun to adjust to it.

Mr. Moderate Anxiety: He stares out the window and is quiet and withdrawn during morning care. At bathtime he complains about the noisy night shift, fusses about the hospital breakfast, and argues that he should be able to sit in the chair and watch TV. Later he apologizes for being a bother, but soon he is complaining of a backache and a headache, "And, by the way, when is that doctor coming back—next year?"

Mrs. Severe Anxiety: She scrutinizes your face as you check her vital signs. "What's my blood pressure now? *Exactly.* Isn't that higher than last time? One point? Two points? Say, is this thing in my arm working? I don't see it dripping. Are you sure? It was going faster yesterday." She examines each pill you give her, turns it over, feels the groove, smells it: "Are you sure this is *my* pill?" She pulls and picks at the covers, "I just can't rest. This bed—I can't stand it much longer. Can't you *do* something, Nurse?"

Mr. Panic: He is scared to death. He jumps each time you approach. His quivering and fidgeting repeatedly set off the monitor alarms. One day he leaps out of bed and, with the IV site dripping blood and the monitor cables flapping behind him, runs frantically down the hall.

Mr. Denial: "Heart attack? That's crazy. That's crazy. Why, back in '89, I had something just like this—one of them hernias. You know, where your stomach crawls up into your chest? I'll be okay, soon's I get home and take some baking soda. Stay in bed for a stomach ache? That's stupid. There's nothing wrong with me."

Mr. Angry: "I've never seen such a bunch of lousy nurses. Why that big fat night nurse, she's so mean! 'No sleeping pills after 5 AM,' she says. Then she jabs me with the dullest needle she can find. And those giggly evening nurses—they just care about their dates and hairdos. That Head Nurse is so high and mighty, she just cares about the equipment—wouldn't notice if I was dead. You better believe I'm never coming back to this dump again! I'll die first."

Mr. Bargainer: "God won't let me die yet. I've got kids to raise. Surely He'll let me finish that. I'll start going to church regularly and give my tithe. Say, Nurse, you sure look nice today. The wife's gonna bring in some candy—you be sure to come by when she's here. You'll be here when I need you, won't you?" He bargains with you or the doctors, but most of all with God.

These are some of the faces of fear that you will see with all their subtle shadings and variations. What do we do about them? Here is a plan that we can put to use in our nursing practice.

1. Watch for the faces of fear. Be alert to the actions and reactions of your individual patients. OBSERVE!

2. Listen to your patients actively, positively.

3. Act as the patients' advocate in helping them deal with their environment, the other members of the health team, their family, and themselves.

This means we are going to do three simple things in helping our patients: observe, listen, and act. To begin, concentrate on *watching*. Everyone you meet, all of your patients—be alert to what they look like, how they express themselves, and how they handle their feelings. Under your nurse's cap (or in place of one), develop antennae that receive patient signals.

Perhaps you have already seen many of the faces of fear. You may have seen the patient who 1. thinks his heart will stop if the monitor stops, 2. thinks interference on the monitor is a sign of heart damage, 3. thinks the monitor's "On" light is a danger signal, 4. is sure that IVs are used only on dying patients, 5. is sure that frequent checks of vital signs mean he's critical, 6. is afraid to have any but the "best" nurses touch him, 7. is afraid to move or turn.

Review 20

You have probably seen other reactions you could add to this list. If so, it's time to proceed to the next skill: *listening*. All of us realize the importance of communicating—we talk *and* listen to our patients. But perhaps we can improve the way we communicate.

Mark with a plus (+) the phrases that you would use in talking with patients. Mark with a zero (0) those you feel shouldn't be used.

____ 1. "You look rather upset."

____ 2. "I know how frightening a hospital can be."

____ 3. "It must be hard to face being inactive."

____ 4. "Of course you'll get well."

____ 5. "Many of our patients feel like you do. I understand how you feel."

____ 6. "It must be difficult to be cooped up in bed."

____ 7. "Come now, let's think about cheerful things."

____ 8. "It must be tough to feel that way."

____ 9. "You'll feel better tomorrow."

____ 10. "It seems to me that you're a little tense and jittery."

____ 11. "You have a good doctor and well-trained nurses. Don't worry."

____ 12. "Would you like to talk about it?"

____ 13. "Now just relax, we'll do the worrying."

____ 14. "We'll watch your monitor, don't you worry about it."

____ 15. "Uh-mm, Oh . . ., Uh huh . . ."

____ 16. "I understand . . ."

Answers and Comments

_+_ 1. Sounds blunt, doesn't it? But if the patient does seem upset, it is an honest opener. He can confirm or deny it. Often he will say, "No, I'm not upset, but I'm sure worried about . . ."

_0_ 2. You don't know how frightening—or painful, or difficult—it is for him. And that is what he really cares about. Try "Hospitals can be frightening."

_+_ 3. "It must be hard to . . ." is a great opener if you finish with words or ideas the patient himself has expressed. If your patient says, "I hate this hospital," you can say, "It must be hard to have to be here and feel that way." Then hang on to your cap, you may hear more than you can comfortably handle. But remember, it's like ventilating a stale-smelling room; the odor will improve.

_0_ 4. Oh yeah? And how do you know? Reassure the patient, don't patronize him. These are adults, not children.

_0_ 5. First you reduce him to just another statistic—one of many—then you play God. If he asks, "Have you ever seen anybody this bad?" try saying "It must be hard to feel so bad."

_+_ 6. "It must be difficult to . . ." is another great opener. It gives the patient the opportunity to evaluate for himself and to let you know.

_0_ 7. One of the best ways to turn your patient into a clam. He will figure you think his thoughts are bad and you don't want to hear nasty things. So he will just shut up.

+   8. "It must be tough to . . ." is as good an opener as those in numbers 3 and 6.

 0   9. And what if he doesn't? What does that make you?

 + 10. An honest reflection of how he looks to you. It tells the patient you are willing to listen to how he *does* feel.

 0 11. So did all the ex-presidents of the United States, and how many of them are alive today? If the patient asks, "What do you think of my doctor?" Give him a *positive,* objective answer. (You can, even if you *can't* stand his doctor!) "He is well-trained," "His patients all do well," "He comes any time you need him," "I like him," "He is my favorite," are all good responses.

 + 12. Excellent! "It" means whatever the patient wants it to mean—an invitation for the patient to select the topic. A good follow-up to numbers 3, 6, and 8. If the patient says, "It sure is tough," you can ask, "Would you like to talk about it?"

 0 13. He would relax if he could. Prompting won't help.

 0 14. Same as 13. Yes, he needs to know you watch the monitor; he should know you can see it from the desk, too. But leave off the "don't worry."

 + 15. Noncommittal, but soothing, comforting sounds. If skillfully used, they show the patient you are listening, not planning tomorrow's dinner. They encourage him to continue without your passing judgment on what he says. Skillful use takes practice; otherwise you sound bored or uncaring.

 0 16. A phrase you should eliminate from your nursing vocabulary. *Nobody* on earth fully understands you, or me, or your patient.

Review 21

Think of the faces of fear you have seen in your patients. What one fear do they all share? Fear of the unknown, right? It's the same fear that makes us cold and sweaty in the dentist's office or at a meeting when we are asked to speak.

What can you do to reduce some of the unknowns surrounding your patient? You do many things consciously and unconsciously. List some of them before you check the list below.

Here are a few of my ideas that might be helpful. Add them to your list if you think they are useful.

Unknown Staff

Introduce yourself to the patient. If you have a name, you are a "person," not just some nurse.

Eliminate unnecessary rotation of assignments among nurses.

Introduce new staff members to the patients.

Unknown Environment

Explain to each patient the things he sees about him. Does he know that the red light on the monitor means that it is "on," not that he is in danger?

Does he think that IVs are only used on the dying?

If the defibrillator must be at his bedside, can you curtain it? Many night nurses remember a patient with bulging eyeballs staring at that "electric chair" machine.

Lack of Orientation to Time and Place

Do you provide a clock and calendar in the unit? No wonder he is confused as to what day or time it is.

Reorient him frequently: "It's 10 AM, and I have a pill for you." "It's 3 PM and I need to see how much is left in your IV bottle."

Does he wear glasses or a hearing aid? What an out-of-focus, frightening world it must be without them.

Unreassuring Reassurances

"You're doing just fine." So why is he still in CCU? Try being specific: "Your pulse is more regular today." "You don't seem short of breath after your bath this morning." "You sat up 15 minutes longer today." Give him tangibles so that he can measure and say to himself, "Yes, I am doing better." The family needs these measuring sticks, too, because they also wonder if he is really improving.

Now we will look at the specific faces of fear to see how we can provide better nursing care for them:

Anxiety can be decreased through activity: Why do you pace the floor or pleat a gum wrapper when you are tense? Since most physical activity is denied these patients, they can at least be allowed a voice in the activities of planning, directing, and choosing what to do when they feel up to it. This gives patients a sense of worth. When we deny them any say in their daily activities, aren't we suggesting that they are mentally as well as physically deficient?

Panic or near-panic often shows itself in abnormally exaggerated ways. Some patients may need the protection of drugs and restraints, but often a "sitter" at the bedside is enough.

Try to see the environment from the patient's point of view. That relaxing seascape may seem a swirling, threatening hurricane to him. The defibrillator or the crash cart may be "a big, black monster." Is his IV threatening to fall and crush him? Does he fly to pieces when you kick the footstool under the bed? If his perceptions are distorted, it may be helpful to reduce the number of stimuli he can respond to.

Denial: Don't contradict him; he only has to deny even harder. Allow him his right to deny, but in small, positive ways emphasize the reality of the situation. You might say things such as: "Your IV must stay in. The monitor still shows us that you may need some medication to help your heart," or "You look tired; may I turn this light off so you can rest?"

Bargaining: Does the patient flatter or compliment you? Maybe he is bargaining with you! Accept this stage and don't rely on his compliments to boost your ego. Then let him move out of the bargaining phase when he is ready. If he has made a bargain with God, the prayer book or rosary that you stuffed in the bottom drawer may be vitally important. His clergyman may be able to give more support than you or the family can offer.

Anger: This is a hard one because anger is often vented on you, the nurse. It helps to remember he is not angry with you; he is mad at what has happened to him.

Possibly some of his anger is justified. After all, hospital staffs aren't perfect. However, it is more likely that the people he rages at are innocent. Battles between staff members and wars between shifts are sometimes started by the patient who is in the anger phase of adjustment. Watch it. If you wage war with this patient's ammunition, you may be shooting a paper cannon.

If the patient is venting his anger on you, understand and try to help others realize that he is angry at fate, or himself, or God—you are just handier.

Your patients will probably wear many masks of fear, changing them frequently. You won't feel lost or helpless if you practice the two phrases: "It must be hard to . . ." and "Would you like to talk about it?"

Mary Bayer, who wrote the poem "Faces of Fear," brings up one other point. "You may be confused by patients who are speaking a 'symbolic' language. You must decode their messages and return your message in *their* code." She tells about a patient lying absolutely rigid, arms beside her, palms up, her eyes rolling back and forth from the wall at her feet, to the wall at her right side and head, to the curtain at her left side. The patient said, "There is a wall at my feet and my head and on both sides of me." Mary replied, "It's too soon for that, isn't it?" The patient began to cry, and said, "I feel like I'm already in my casket." By using the patient's symbolic language, Mary helped her voice her fears.

Last, don't try to force your patient from one phase to the next. He moves at his own speed, and you must move with him. If you don't stifle the mechanisms or hopes of each phase, you will provide your patient with real psychological support.

Alterations in Comfort (p. 21)

Review 22

Euphemisms help nurses and doctors cope. "Pt. c/o being uncomfortable." "Pt. c/o discomfort." These patients are in *pain!* They hurt. And some of the procedures we do cause more pain.

1. Disease processes that cause pain include _____ _____ and
   _____.

   myocardial ischemia
   pericarditis

2. Pain can cause a sympathetic nervous system response that increases myocardial
   _____ _____ .

   oxygen consumption

3. If a painful procedure is scheduled, it helps to give the patient analgesia _____ minutes before.

   30

4. Patients on a neuromuscular blocking agent (eg, Pavulon) do/do not) feel pain.

   do

5. Pavulon is used to help _____ the patient's breathing with the respirator.

   synchronize

6. The patient on Pavulon can be fully _____. (Think how terrifying this could be!)

   conscious

7. Three things you can do for this patient: _____, _____ _____, _____.

   sedation   pain control
       reassurance

EMERGENCY AND RESUSCITATIVE TREATMENT (p. 22)

Review 23

Cardiopulmonary Resuscitation (p. 22)

1. Two certificates *all* CCU staff should have (and keep current) are: _____ and _____.

   ACLS   CPR

Defibrillation (p. 22)

1. You recognize ventricular fibrillation on the monitor. You check the patient _____. If he is unconscious and has no pulses, you use the _____ immediately. (You do NOT call the supervisor. You do NOT wait for a doctor's order. If you do, your patient is dead.)

   immediately   defibrillator

Assisted Ventilation (p. 22)

The respiratory therapists won't always be in the CCU. So talk to them when they are there; find out what you need to know or do. If you need more help, ask if you can spend some time in their department. You will find they will be happy to teach you when you show interest in their specialty. (After all, the patient who can't breathe is going to be just as dead as the one whose heart stops.)

COMMUNICATION (p. 22)

Review 24

Have you ever been a patient? Or a close relative or friend of a patient? Weren't you desperate for explanations and answers? Communication—that is what you needed. And in the CCU, you, the nurse, are the prime communicator. There are four areas of communication.

1. Patient and family. You need to explain, explain, _____. (They aren't going to remember, their stress level is too high.)

   explain

2. You are the _____ between the doctor, patient, and family.

   liaison

3. You must keep the _____ posted on any significant change in the patient's condition.   doctor

4. _____ during and between shifts are vital. We have all heard, "Well, the other shift didn't tell me." In the CCU that could be a death sentence for poor Mr. Kardiak.   Reports

COLLECTION AND RECORDING OF DATA (pp. 22–23)

Review 25

1. As with other patients, as soon as possible, you obtain a _____ _____ on the patient.   nursing history

2. You establish a baseline _____ _____.   nursing diagnosis

3. You develop and institute a _____ _____ _____.   nursing care plan

4. Specific to the CCU, you record an admission _____ _____ and you further _____ all changes.   monitor strip
document

5. You will also find that your CCU protocol will specify _____ intervals when you will run monitor strips.   regular

6. Subsequent chapters will discuss drug therapy and nursing notes in detail so let's move on to:

EDUCATION (pp. 23–27)

Review 26

When you become a CCU nurse it is your privilege and responsibility to help teach others: students, staff nurses, patients, and family.

1. Formal teaching is usually _____ attempted during the acute phases.   not

2. Then it is most important simply to _____ _____.   answer questions

3. Most patients and families have many misconceptions about heart disease, treatment and recovery. One of your main teaching objectives will be to _____ these misconceptions.   correct

4. It is important to _____ information and to give _____ information to patient and family. (I remember when my husband was discharged after a suspected MI. Together, we listened carefully to the discharge instructions. When we got home it was obvious we had heard different instructions!)   repeat   written

5. You may have hospital brochures and American Association of Critical Care Nurses' brochures. Don't forget the American Heart Association has excellent brochures too.

3

Monitoring in the Coronary Care Unit

Welcome to the fascinating world of monitors! Chapter 3 basically introduces you to the equipment. There are some terms used in this chapter that will be explained in much greater detail in later chapters. But if you are not familiar with them and you are wondering what you are missing, let's do a little review.

Review 1

Label Figure 3.1 showing the electrical system of the heart.

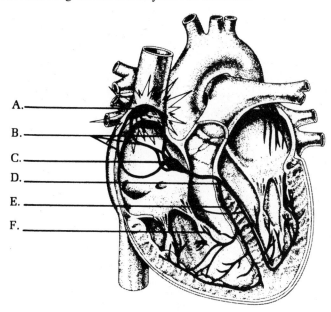

A. SA node

B. Internodal tracts

C. AV node

D. Bundle of His

E. Right and left bundle branches

F. Purkinje fibers

Figure 3.1

How did you do? If you made any mistakes, don't worry, you will have this in greater detail later. Now let's see if you have a very basic understanding of the conduction system.

Review 2

1. The normal pacemaker of the heart is in the _____ node.

   sinoatrial (SA)

2. The SA node normally discharges an electrical force _____ to _____ times per minute.

   60   100

3. Right now (if you are normal), your heart rate is being controlled by the _____ _____.

   SA node

4. Your heart rate is probably between _____ and _____.

   60   100

5. The electrical impulse leaves the SA node and travels through the _____ _____, _____ _____, _____ _____ _____, _____ _____ and _____ _____, and finally stimulates the cells at the Purkinje-myocardial junction to discharge their stored electrical forces, causing a ventricular contraction.

   internodal tracts
   AV node   Bundle of His
   bundle branches   Purkinje fibers

6. The discharge of electrical forces causing this contraction is called _____.

   depolarization

7. After depolarization, the rest or recovery period is called _____. (If you have trouble with this, associate the *re* in *re*polarization with *rest* or *recovery*.)

   repolarization

8. The pacemaking function of the SA node can be taken over by an _____ pacemaker.

   ectopic

9. The various phases of the cardiac cycle can be identified on an _____.

   ECG

10. The electrocardiogram records the _____ forces from the heart that are transmitted to the body's surface.

    electrical

11. Identify which is the machine and which is the printed record.
    A. Electrocardiogram: _____
    B. Electrocardiograph: _____

    record
    machine

    (Just remember tele*graph*/tele*gram*. Now, if you've got that, let's use ECG for both machine and record—it's so much easier!)

Perhaps you are wondering why the monitor pattern goes up and down (positive and negative) and why it changes with different leads on the monitor or ECG. Does Figure 3.2 explain that?

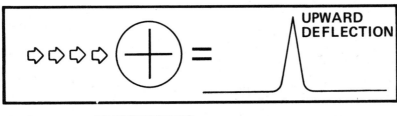

CURRENT FLOW   **ELECTRODES**

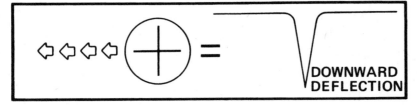

Figure 3.2. Current flowing *toward* a positive electrode causes a positive inflection. Current flowing *away* from a positive electrode causes a negative deflection.

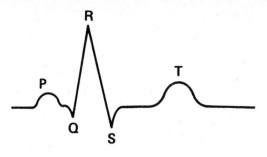
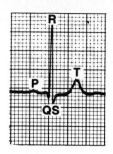

Figure 3.3. Normal cardiac cycle.   **Figure 3.4**

Review 3

You will meet up with the terms P, Q, R, S, T in this chapter (there is a lot more in Chapter 8). Figure 3.3 is the artist's drawing of this (the cardiac cycle) and Figure 3.4 is the real thing from the monitor strip.

1. For Chapter 3 you only need to know that the P wave shows depolarization of the
   _____.   atria

2. The R wave shows depolarization of the _____.   ventricles

3. The ST segment can be depressed or elevated and that indicates myocardial _____.   ischemia

4. In Chapter 4 you will be introduced to the Q wave significance. For now, just identify the Q wave on the figures.

Review 4

Chapter 3 mentions lead II, MCL$_1$, V leads, etc, terms you will thoroughly cover in Chapter 8. If you are perplexed over these, let's simply say:

12-lead ECG:
    3 standard, bipolar, limb leads = I, II, III
    3 modified, augmented, unipolar leads = aVR, aVL, and aVF
    6 chest (precordial) unipolar leads = V$_1$, V$_2$, V$_3$, V$_4$, V$_5$, V$_6$

Now the monitor: lead II (comparable to ECG lead II). MCL$_1$ is equivalent to V$_1$ and so is called Modified Chest lead 1. If you must know more, sneak a peak at the figures in Chapter 8. But don't get bogged down in details yet.

Review 5

1. The success of CCU depends on the nurse's ability to detect _____ and   warning
   _____ arrhythmias and to _____ them immediately.   lethal   treat

2. Originally, _____ monitoring was of prime importance.   cardiac

3. Now _____ monitoring is equally important.   hemodynamic

4. Number 3 is very important in patients with advanced _____ _____.   heart failure

5. Continuous monitoring of the patient's oxygenation status can be done with pulse
   _____ and _____.   oximetry   S$\bar{v}o_2$

6. The data gathered by nurses and staff can be integrated in a _____ _____   clinical information
   _____.   system

CARDIAC MONITORING (p. 29)

Review 6

1. In the "normal" heart, the _____ node located in the _____ _____ discharges an _____ stimulus that spreads through the _____ system to stimulate the _____ to _____.

   sinoatrial   right atrium
   electrical   conduction
   myocardium   contract

2. This _____ force spreads outward from the heart to the _____ _____ where _____ attached to the skin can _____ the electrical signals.

   electrical   body
   surface   electrodes   detect

3. The cardiac _____ picks up the electrical signals and displays them on an _____ (commonly known as the _____) as a continuous ECG.

   monitor
   oscilloscope   monitor

4. You, the nurse, can _____ the ECG wave forms and identify _____ (or base-line), or any changes in cardiac _____, _____, or _____. (Those last three phrases are part of the gospel of the CCU; you will learn much more about them very soon.)

   analyze   normal
   rate   rhythm   conduction

MONITORING EQUIPMENT (pp. 29–30)

Now let's make friends with the monitor. There are two maxims I would like to pass on to you. The first is original; the second came from a Basic Nursing instructor long before the advent of monitoring. First, the monitor is your slave; you are its master. And second, you need to be more intelligent or more stubborn than your equipment. There will be times when you will need mastery, intelligence, and tenacity. You will also need practice. So, let's take a look at the equipment.

Review 7

1. _____ are the little thingamigigs you are going to attach to the patient's chest.

   Electrodes

2. The electrical impulses that the electrodes pick up must be transmitted to the monitor by _____ _____.

   lead wires

3. These connect into the _____ _____.

   patient cable

4. The patient cable has a _____ on one end for the lead wires and the other end plugs into the _____.

   receptacle
   monitor

5. The monitor has several jobs. One part of it _____ the original electrical impulses (by about 1,000!).

   amplifies

6. A magnetic field, called a _____, creates the wave forms you see on the monitor.

   galvanometer

7. Those wave forms are displayed for you on the screen which is called an _____ screen.

   oscilloscopic

8. In actual practice, numbers 5, 6, and 7 will simply be known as the _____ (as in, "Hey, look at the monitor! What's he doing now?).

   monitor

9. You can adjust _____, _____, and _____ of the monitor picture. (That's better than TV.)

   size   position   brightness

10. Some monitors can display two ECG leads at once; they are called _____ channels.

    dual

11. The monitor counts the _____ waves.

    R

12. These are the electrical waves from ventricular _____.

    depolarization

13. They are NOT from ventricular _____. Go back to the introduction of this chapter if you are confused.

    contraction

14. Integrated with the rate meter is an _____ system which warns if the patient's heart rate _____ _____ the limits which you set.

    alarm
    falls outside

15. By setting a range (eg, 50 to 120) you will be warned if the patient's heart rate is _____ than 50 or _____ than 120.

less   greater

16. Will the preset range always be 50 to 120? _____

No

17. Identifying things as they flit by on the monitor is tough. So the monitor can provide a permanent _____ record of what you may (or may not) have seen.

printed

18. What are you trying to identify on Mr. Kardiak's monitor? _____ _____ _____

Early warning signs

19. These are arrhythmias that if not treated could lead to _____ arrhythmias.

lethal

20. Some monitors can _____ their picture for your closer observation.

freeze

21. Some monitors have _____ systems that can play back the preceeding 5 to 60 seconds.

memory

22. If you are buying new equipment, which would you opt for?_____

_____

_____

_____

THE OPERATION OF CARDIAC MONITORS (pp. 30–34)

Review 8

Let's use our heads (we don't need them for caps anymore!) You have a monitor up there on the wall or on a cart and a patient lying over there on the bed. How to connect them?

1. Obviously, you need _____ on the patient's chest.

electrodes

2. Then, connecting or _____ wires from the electrodes to the junction box on the patient _____.

lead
cable

3. And the other end of the patient cable connects to the _____.

monitor

4. The monitor connects to electricity through a _____ cable.

monitor

5. You need to adjust the _____ to get the best picture.

monitor

6. You need to set _____ and _____ alarms.

high   low

Electrodes and Their Attachment (pp. 30–31)
Review 9

1. Look at them closely. Little discs that are prepackaged, disposable, and probably _____.

pregelled

2. The gel is a _____ medium that provides the necessary space between electrode and skin.

conductive

3. This helps reduce _____ interference at the skin surface.

electrical

4. Pregelled electrodes should remain moist and not _____ the skin.

irritate

Location of Electrodes (pp. 31–33)
Review 10

1. Your CCU may use _____, 4, or 5 electrodes.

3

2. This depends on the number of _____ _____ your patient cables accommodate and if your monitors are _____ or _____ channel.

lead wires
single   dual

3. Let's start with the simplest: three electrodes. One electrode is a _____ to carry off extraneous electrical activity.

ground

4. _____ of the electrodes detect the heart's electrical activity.

Two

29

5. Newer equipment may use up to _____ electrodes for multiple ECG views.

6. The two most common three-lead views are _____ and _____ (modified chest lead I). (These will be explained more in later chapters, don't worry about them now.)

7. Lead II is especially useful for identifying _____.

8. You can quickly attach a lead II in an emergency by saying to yourself, "Cross the heart. High on the _____, low on the _____."

9. That is, the right electrode goes to the right of the _____, below the _____.

10. The left electrode goes at the lowest _____ that you can palpate and on the _____ _____ line.

11. The ground electrode goes on the right lower _____ _____.

12. With lead II you will be monitoring electrical activity coming from the _____ to the _____ electrode.

13. This lead gives you the tallest _____ wave.

14. In monitoring the course of an MI, lead _____ shows the ST segment best. (You will learn more later about why it is important to monitor the ST segment.)

15. For an MCL₁ place the right electrode in the _____ interspace at the right border of the _____.

16. Place the left electrode near the left _____ just under the outer portion of the _____.

17. The ground electrode can go in the right _____ area.

	5
	II MCL₁
	arrhythmias
	right left
	sternum clavicle
	rib
	anterior axillary
	rib cage
	right
	left
	R
	MCL₁
	4th
	sternum
	shoulder
	clavicle
	shoulder

Attachment of Electrode to Skin (pp. 33–34)
Review 11

1. In order to get a good monitor picture, you must do a good job of _____ the electrodes.

2. After you select the electrode sites, you will probably need to _____ a 4-inch area for each electrode on Mr. Kardiak.

3. Then cleanse the area with _____, rubbing well.

4. Be sure you thoroughly _____ the areas.

5. It is best to connect the _____ _____ to the electrodes before you apply them to the patient.

6. Most electrodes now used are pregelled. Don't open them ahead of time; they will _____ _____.

7. Avoid squishing the gel out by _____ _____ _____ on the gelled area.

8. You suspect that the electrodes need to be changed if the monitor picture is less _____, or it looks like the skin may become _____.

9. A considerable shifting of electrode position will change the monitor pattern; you would want to run a _____ and _____ strip if that happened.

	attaching
	shave
	alcohol
	dry
	lead wires
	dry out
	pressing too hard
	distinct irritated
	before after

Connecting the Wires from the Electrodes to the Monitor (p. 34)
Review 12

1. The _____ _____ carries signals from the patient to the monitor.

2. The _____ cable carries electrical power from the wall socket to the monitor.

	patient cable
	monitor

3. The openings on the receptacle (sometimes called a junction box) on a three-wire patient cable will be marked _____ or _____, _____ or _____, and _____ or _____.

R RA
L LA G RL

4. Lead II: simply insert the lead wire from each electrode into the _____ opening on the receptacle.

corresponding

5. For MCL$_1$, you _____ the wires. That is, you put the _____ electrode lead wire into the _____ opening.

reverse right
left

6. And the _____ electrode wire goes into the _____ opening. But, please, put the _____ wire into the G opening.

left right
ground

7. When all connections are secure, pin the _____ _____ _____ to the patient's gown.

patient cable receptacle

8. Don't forget to insert the patient cable into the cable socket on the _____.

monitor

Adjusting the Monitor *(p. 34)*
Review 13

1. You should be able to adjust your monitor pattern for _____.

brightness

2. You should also be able to _____ the pattern and adjust the _____ of the wave forms.

center height

3. This is necessary in order for the monitor to count the _____ waves and thus the heart rate.

R

Setting the Alarm System *(p. 34)*
Review 14

1. You establish the _____ and _____ rate alarms based on the patient's heart rate.

high low

2. Your CCU may prescribe a "normal" range." *The Manual* suggests _____ to _____.

50 140

3. False alarms (usually caused by patient movement) may tempt you to _____ _____ the alarm. Don't!

turn
off

Review 15

Now let's put it all together with a Monitor Game that takes you step by step through the procedure for applying a monitor. Practice on yourself, a cohort, a patient, or even a pillow if you have to. You lose five points if your first monitored patient asks, "Is this the first time you've done this?"

Points

1. Find a monitor that you can practice on. (In some hospitals this should be worth more than one point.)

(1)

2. Got the instruction manual? Then read it.

(1)

3. Plug the power cord into the monitor. (Look again. It plugs in somewhere.)

(1)

4. You need a patient cable to run from the monitor to your patient. Attach it to the monitor. (Check the instruction manual.)

(5)

5. Where are the patient leads that connect the cable to the patient's electrodes? (They may or may not already be attached to the electrodes.) You should find three skinny wires that plug into a connector on the free end of the cable. (Five points when you can plug them in without fumbling.)

(5)

6. Now look at your electrodes. They are usually prepackaged. You say Central Supply will kill you if you open too many for practice? Then try to get some accidentally opened ones or one set just for practice. Read the instructions. You must attach the lead wires to the skin electrodes. Do you need conductive jelly, paste, or are the electrodes "pre-gooped"?

(5)

7. Where do the electrodes go on the patient? Let's do a lead II. Say to yourself: "Cross your heart. One high on the right, one low on the left." The ground electrode goes on the lower right rib cage. (5)

   A. Shave the patient, if necessary. Clean the area with alcohol and dry. (5)

   B. Connect electrodes to wires. (5)

   C. Put "goop" on the electrodes, if needed. (5)

   D. Attach electrodes to the patient. (5)

(*Note:* You can do D before B, but some patients complain that it hurts when you snap (push hard) the electrode wires into the electrode pads on their chest. Try it on yourself both ways.)

8. Now step back and admire your work. What? No monitor picture?

   A. Did you give the machine time to warm up? (1)

   B. Is the plug in the wall socket? (1)

   C. Is the cable plugged into the monitor? (1)

   D. Is the patient cable in place? (1)

   E. Are the wires on the cable firmly inserted into the connector? (1)

   F. Are the electrodes on the wire? (1)

   G. Are the electrodes on the patient? (1)

   H. All right—did you turn the monitor on? (1)

9. Is there a Sensitivity or Gain dial on your machine? Try it. See what it does. (1)

10. How about a Position Selector switch? Try it, too. (1)

11. Too much electrical interference? (The ECG pattern looks like a satin stitch on the sewing machine—60 little lines per second.) You have to get rid of any interference.

   A. Sometimes just changing to a different wall outlet will help.

   B. If not, call your engineer to check the outlet. No engineer? Ask your ECG technician how they eliminate interference. No ECG technician? Find the monitor salesman (often a very helpful person).

   C. If you are monitoring with a portable monitor where interference is a problem, it is often necessary to plug a ground wire into the back of the monitor. The other end of this ground wire has an "alligator clip" (it looks like jaws and is capable of biting); you attach this to a water pipe. Try using the radiator if there are no water lines.

12. Find the rate meter. It's like a computer that shows heart rate at all times. See if it's accurate. All you have to do is check the rate on the meter and compare it with the patient's radial pulse. If they are not the same, believe your watch; someone may have fiddled with the rate meter. (2)

13. Find the Low-Rate Alarm. Set it around 50. (2)

14. Find the High-Rate Alarm. Set it about 20 points above the patient's pulse rate. Scratch the electrodes with your finger or have the patient wiggle in bed. How does this affect the ECG pattern? Does it do anything to the counter and alarms? (2)

15. Try the "beeper" (volume) on and off, loud and soft. Do you think that beep-per-beat might bother your patient? (It would me.) (2)

16. Identify any other switch, knob, light, lever, or dial, and try it out. (One point for each.)

Scoring
55—How come YOU aren't writing this?
50—When I have my MI, will you be my nurse?
45—You can do better.
40—You *better* do better.
Below 40—Anything would be better. Practice makes perfect.

PROBLEMS WITH CARDIAC MONITORING *(pp. 35–37)*

Review 16

1. The rate meter is not all that intelligent. It counts all _____ deflections as heartbeats.

    upward

2. Muscle _____ can be interpreted by the monitor as heartbeats. (Just watch what happens when the patient brushes his teeth! See Fig. 3–5 in *The Manual.*)

    contractions

3. You try to eliminate this interference by NOT placing electrodes directly over _____ _____.

    large muscles

4. Low-rate alarms can result whenever any part of the monitor system becomes _____ (see Fig. 3–6 in *The Manual*).

    loose

5. A flat line on the monitor is NOT ventricular standstill if the patient is sitting up and talking to you. Treat the _____, not the monitor.

    patient

6. Low-rate alarms can be triggered by R waves that are too _____ (see Fig. 3–7 in *The Manual*).

    short

7. Remember that you can increase the _____ of the complexes by adjusting a control on the monitor.

    amplitude

8. Sometimes _____ the leads is necessary to give the monitor something it can count.

    changing

9. Once you have seen electrical interference you will probably recognize it (see Fig. 3–8 in *The Manual*). It's a series of _____ spikes per second.

    60

10. To troubleshoot electrical interference you first make sure that all connecting wires are _____ _____ _____.

    firmly in place

11. If you can't correct the interference, you may need an electrical engineer to check for improper _____.

    grounding

12. Does this matter? _____

    Yes!

13. Leakage current and improper grounding can combine to kill a patient. It works like this: If Mr. Kardiak has a transvenous pacemaker, leakage current from the _____ may travel via the _____ _____ to his heart and induce _____ _____.

    monitor   pacing catheter   ventricular fibrillation

14. Nurses on nightshift will often see a wandering baseline (see Fig. 3–9 in *The Manual*). This is usually caused by _____.

    respirations

15. Try to _____ the pattern on the monitor so alarms aren't triggered and let the patient sleep.

    center

16. Sometimes _____ will have to be moved off the lower ribs to correct a wandering baseline.

    electrodes

17. Check the patient's skin carefully for _____. (While he's awake, please!)

    irritation

Review 17

The care and understanding of monitors is almost like the care and understanding of children. Experience helps. I will introduce you to Nurse Old Pro and the nurse she is orienting, Nurse Neo Phyte. Maybe we can learn from their experience.

    Suppose we visit them on the night shift. Old Pro is relaxing in front of a console containing five flickering monitors. Four of the patients are visible in the open unit and one is a convalescent patient in an adjoining room with only his monitor visible. Pro's eyes constantly scan the monitors in front of her.

Pro: Such a quiet night—I'm afraid you won't see much.

Neo: Oh, look at monitor 1. Is that heart block? Shall I call the doctor?

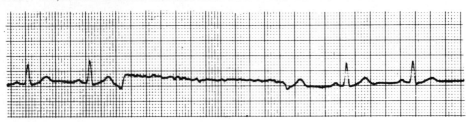

Figure 3.5

Pro: No, hold on a minute. The first two and the last two complexes are perfectly normal. That squiggly line across the middle doesn't look like it comes from the heart. Notice that sharp V right after the second complex: there is no reason for a pattern to jump up like that. Why don't you go and check the patient's electrodes?

Neo: (checks and returns) One electrode was loose. I taped it down and now he's normal again.

Pro: Too bad we can't patent your method of making people normal. Incidentally, anything on the monitor that is not caused by the heart's action is called an "artifact."

Neo: Oh dear, 2 is going from the top to the bottom of the monitor. That's not right. Does he have a loose electrode, too?

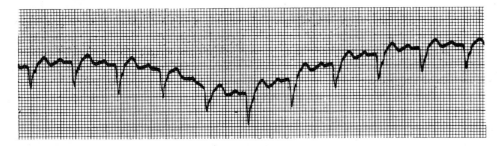

Figure 3.6

Pro: That's a pattern I like to see. I will bet you a cup of coffee that he's snoring. That's a respiratory deflection. There are some abnormal things about his pattern, but the "hills and valleys" cycles are just fine. If you want to get rid of them you just reposition the chest electrodes. But let's not awaken him.

Neo: Will I ever learn when to panic?

Pro: (laughing) Of course you will. And I'll tell you a secret. Even the pros panic; we just make good use of that extra adrenalin. Now, don't panic, but I would like you to check 3. I can still see a regular pattern, but something's going on. I'm just not sure what's causing it.

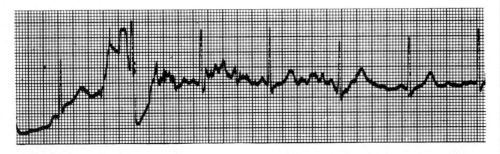

Figure 3.7

Neo: (returns after several minutes) He was scratching! The electrode jelly makes him itch. I washed his chest off and moved the electrodes a bit.

Pro: That's good. Now what on earth is happening next door on monitor 5? (High-rate alarm sounds.)

Neo: (racing for patient's room) I'll go see!

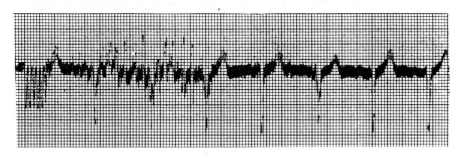

Figure 3.8

Pro: (to herself) It's electrical interference, but why suddenly in the middle of the night?

Neo: (returns shaking her head) He couldn't sleep, so do you know what he was doing? Shaving with an electric razor!

Pro: Look at those closely spaced lines on his monitor strip. There are actually 60 of them per second. That's 60-cycle electrical interference.

Neo: I don't think I'll count them. By the way, I told the patient that we didn't think it was safe for him to shave with a razor that plugs in the wall. I promised to bring the unit's battery-operated razor in the morning.

Pro: Good. We have to be really careful about shock hazards in the CCU, especially in patients with transvenous pacemakers.

Neo: Why did the high-rate alarm go off on this patient?

Pro: Look at the strip: the monitor counts all upright lines. It tried to count all the 60-cycle interference, so it exceeded the high-alarm setting. I've got the high set on 110.

Neo: There is so much to learn; how will I know the real thing? I'll probably defibrillate a patient for interference.

Pro: You'll know. I think I'll go get a cup of coffee; I'll be right back. (leaves)

Neo: (A few seconds later the alarm rings on monitor 4.) Oh dear, oh look! That's it— I'm sure its *ventricular fibrillation!* What do I do? I remember—check the patient. (runs to bedside) Mr. Four? Mr. Four? Why don't you answer? No pulse, none. Keep cool. Push the emergency alarm. (Alarm sounds outside the unit.) Get the defibrillator.

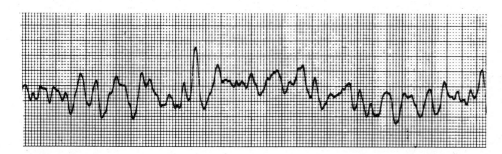

Figure 3.9

Pro: (races in to answer alarm, looks at patient) Aha, you knew! Good girl. Go ahead, defibrillate him—quickly.

Did you pick up a few ideas on the causes and cures of interference? When you are thoroughly familiar with normal rhythm and arrhythmias, interference will be easy to spot.

COMPUTERIZED ARRHYTHMIA MONITORING *(pp. 38–40)*

I remember when the salesperson brought that new-fangled computer monster into our CCU. Those of us who were old-fashioned CCU nurses sniffed skeptically, but soon we were avidly playing with our latest toy. Is computerized arrhythmia monitoring the answer? I don't know. Does your hospital have it? If so, go get acquainted. If not, let's review the principles involved anyway.

Review 18

1. A high percentage of serious arrhythmias go undetected in CCUs. (True/False) — True

2. In theory, a computer can be programmed to recognize _____ or _____ and to identify _____. — normal abnormal arrhythmias

3. The computer's alarm can be programmed so it will "ring" and also _____ _____ _____ _____. — run a rhythm strip

4. The computer can show a continual _____ report and also present an _____ trend. — status hourly

5. Are the computers foolproof? _____ — No! Artifacts fool computers, too.

6. The computerized monitors' advantage is that they don't get _____, they don't daydream, and they don't need coffee breaks. — fatigued

7. A conventional monitor alarms for _____ or _____ arrhythmias. Computerized monitors can be programmed to detect other _____ arrhythmias. — fast slow warning

COMPUTERIZED ST-SEGMENT MONITORING *(p. 41)*

Review 19

You have been briefly introduced to the importance of the ST-segment. (More in Chapter 15 of *The Manual.*)

1. If the ST-segment is elevated or depressed it can mean myocardial _____. — ischemia

2. ST-segment monitoring may be part of a _____ monitor system, and/or the nurse may do it by analyzing the monitor strips. — multi-channel

3. The lead with the _____ R wave is best for ST-segment monitoring. — highest

TELEMETRY *(p. 41)*

Review 20

A Candy Striper (high-school volunteer) came flying down the hall and nearly crash-landed on the desk. "That man—the one with the thing around his neck that makes his heart beat—one of those little wires came off . . . Hurry, he's going to die!"

Just what was she so upset about? The poor panicky Candy Striper misunderstood the function of telemetric monitoring. And so do many other people.

The CCU nurse needs to understand telemetry well enough to be able to apply it and to explain it to the patient, family, and others.

Review 21

Let's go over the components of telemetry and see how well you could explain it. Pretend you are talking with your patient, Mr. Kardiak, as you prepare to transfer him out of CCU. Complete the following statements, then check them against my suggestions.

You: Mr. Kardiak, I'm going to put a telemetry set-up on you so that we can continue monitoring you after you move out of CCU.

Mr Kardiak: You don't say? What are you sticking those things on me for?

You: These electrode pads on your chest _____ _____ _____.

pick up the electrical signals that come from your heart

Mr Kardiak: Hmm, what do those little wires do?

You: The electrode wires _____ _____ _____.

carry the signals to this little box that you will wear around your neck

Mr Kardiak: That thing you're putting around my neck . . . what's it do?

You: This little box that you will be wearing is a _____. It will _____ _____.

transmitter   send your heart's pattern back to the ICCU station as radio waves

Mr Kardiak: How about that! What makes it work?

You: There is a _____ inside this box that keeps it operating.

battery

Mr Kardiak: Great. What happens to the signals after they reach the nurses' station?

You: We see them on a _____ in CCU.

monitor

Mr Kardiak: Really? You mean, even though I'm out of sight, in the CCU you can still see my heart?

You: That's right. The CCU nurses will _____ _____.

keep a close watch on how your heart behaves

Mr Kardiak: That's kinda comforting to know.

You: If the _____ or _____ become loose, we will have to come in and fix them because this will cause too much interference in the pattern that the CCU nurses are seeing. So if we have to bother you in the middle of the night, we are apologizing in advance.

electrodes   wires

Mr Kardiak: No sweat. I'm used to you folks waking me up.

You: Now, I want to be sure you understand that telemetry only shows up a pattern like an ECG of your heart's activity. It does not _____ _____. So there's no danger if you become unhooked. OK?

control (or affect) how your heart beats

Mr Kardiak: Yeah, I got that straight. But can I get a shock from this?

You: No, it does not conduct any electricity from the battery to you. So you can't _____. (The next day you ask Mr. Kardiak if he has any questions.)

get a shock from it

Mr Kardiak: I sure do. During the night they came in and switched these little things on my chest all around. What were they doing?

You: They changed the position of the electrodes to get a different _____ _____ _____ _____. The pattern they were seeing wasn't clear enough. It's similar to your TV set—sometimes one channel comes in better than the others. I guess you could say that they switched channels on your "TV" to get a clearer picture of your heart.

picture of your heart

INVASIVE HEMODYNAMIC MONITORING *(pp. 41–47)*

Review 22

The cardiac monitor gives us a continuous picture of the heart's activity. But our real concern is the "work" the heart is accomplishing as part of a closed, pressurized circulatory system. Is the left ventricular muscle contracting adequately? Is the heart able to pump out all the blood it receives? Is the treatment we are using helping? Measuring the

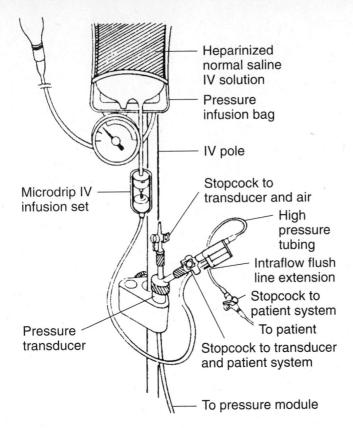

Figure 3.10. Hemodynamic monitoring set-up with transducer flush system.

pressures in the heart chambers could help answer those questions. In the early days of CCU we could only check the systemic blood pressure and the central venous pressure.

1. Central venous pressure catheters can measure only _____ atrium and _____ _____ _____ pressure.

   right   superior vena cava

2. Normal CVP ranges from _____ to _____ cm H₂O.

   5   10

3. But in a patient with impaired cardiac function, we would really like to measure (and assist) the performance of the (right/left) ventricle.

   left

4. This patient's left ventricle (can/cannot) pump out all the blood it receives with each beat.

   cannot

5. Thus the volume and pressure in the left ventricle is greater than normal at the end of the filling period, which is called _____.

   diastole

6. Using some of the initials that CCU people love, we say there is an increase in _____.

   LVEDP

7. Make sure you've got that; spell it out: _____ _____ _____ _____.

   left ventricular end-diastolic pressure

Review 23

Before we go further with pressures, let's take a look at the parts of this system for hemodynamic monitoring.

1. A pressure _____ converts the waves from the catheter to something you can interpret on the patient's pressure monitor.

   transducer

2. The transducer is connected by a fluid-filled _____ _____ tubing to the pulmonary artery catheter.

   high pressure

3. It is important that the high-pressure tubing be short—not over _____ inches.

48

4. You would prime the system with a _____ flush solution.

heparin

5. You maintain a continuous flush of about _____ to _____ mL/hr.

3 5

6. Now take a look at the transducer's all-important position: it must be level with the patient's _____ _____.

right atrium

7. This reference point is called the _____ _____.

phlebostatic axis

8. To find this site, draw one imaginary line down the _____ line and another from the _____ intercostal space. Where they intersect is the _____ _____.

midaxillary
4th
phlebostatic axis

9. Your patient's bed can be adjusted from 0 to _____° as long as you keep the _____ at the phlebostatic axis and you won't affect the accuracy of your readings.

60
transducer

10. Remember though that if your patient turns to a _____ position, especially the _____ lateral, the readings will be inaccurate.

lateral
left

Review 24

Now let's follow the pulmonary artery catheter into the heart. Figure 3–14 in *The Manual* is excellent. Also our Figures 3.11 to 3.14 show the catheter being inserted and the pressure recordings you would see on the monitor (we will cover those pressures in detail shortly).

1. Pulmonary artery catheters can have from _____ to _____ lumens.

2 5

2. One mm from the distal tip is a small _____.

balloon

3. The balloon is _____ for the initial insertion.

deflated

4. The catheter is inserted through the _____ (arm) vein and advanced to the _____ _____ _____.

antecubital
superior vena cava

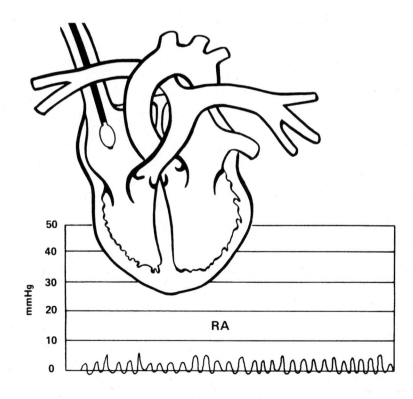

The normal right atrium is pretty much a low-pressure system. The pressure recordings seen on the monitor are minimal, similar to this and below 10 mm Hg.

Figure 3.11. The right atrium.

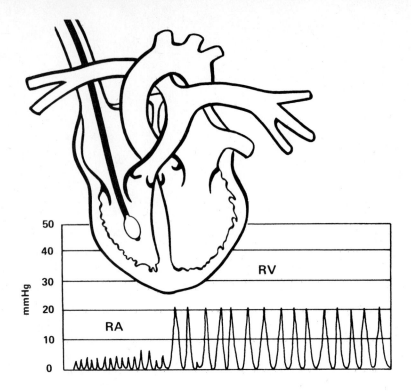

Figure 3.12. The right ventricle.

The inflated balloon helps the catheter to float as it is advanced into the right ventricle.

The normal right ventricular pressure is 20/5. (Compare that to the systemic pressure of 130/70.)

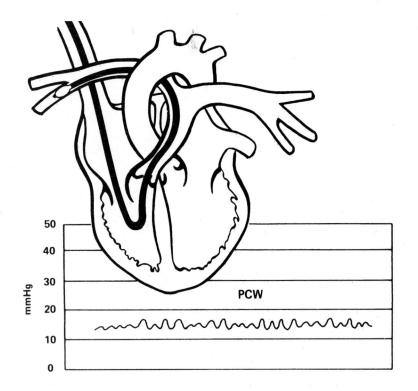

Figure 3.13. Pulmonary capillary wedge pressure.

The catheter, with balloon inflated, is advanced until it wedges in a small branch of the pulmonary artery. Normal capillary wedge pressure ranges from 5 to 12 mm Hg.

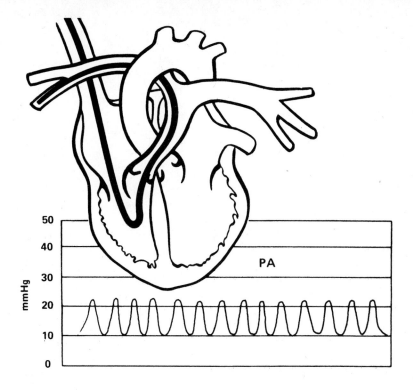

Figure 3.14. Pulmonary artery pressure.

With the balloon deflated the normal PAP is 25/10. Diastolic pressure is used to assess left ventricular function.

5. Then the balloon is inflated and it "floats" the catheter through the right atrium and _____ _____ and into a _____ _____.

    right ventricle
    pulmonary artery

6. When the balloon reaches a small enough artery that it can go no farther, it stays there and that is called the _____ _____ _____ _____.

    pulmonary capillary wedge position

7. Now, use the initials and we won't have to spell that out anymore: _____.

    PCWP

8. Leave the balloon inflated and take a pressure reading (our Figure 3.13). This is the _____ pressure.

    PCWP

9. PCWP measures the pressure in the pulmonary _____ bed.

    capillary

10. And (the important point) this reflects the _____. (Use initials, please.)

    LVEDP

11. Look at Figure 3–14 in *The Manual* and let's get a clear idea of what's happening in the cardiopulmonary circulation and what you are trying to measure.

12. Let's back up: The left ventricle does not empty completely, so the left _____ meets with resistance and higher pressure when it tries to empty into the left ventricle.

    atrium

13. Therefore, when the blood tries to empty into the _____ _____, the pulmonary circulation meets with increased pressure.

    left atrium

14. The pressure and congestion in the pulmonary veins backs up into the pulmonary _____.

    capillaries

15. And you have just measured that with your _____. (Aren't you proud of yourself?)

    PCWP

16. What might happen if you left the balloon inflated? ____ _____ _____

    a pulmonary embolus

17. So, deflate the balloon and take a pressure reading: now you can take the _____ _____ systolic and diastolic pressures.

    pulmonary artery

18. Matter of fact, the monitor will give you a _____ reading of pulmonary artery pressures.

    continuous

19. What else can this "sophisticated" catheter do? Well, take a look at Figure 3–17 in *The Manual*. See the right atrial port and the venous infusion port? With the catheter in place these will be in the _____ _____. (Naturally!)   right atrium

20. The right atrial port allows you to measure _____ _____ pressure.   right atrial

21. And now you can administer _____ _____ into the right atrium.   IV fluids

22. Now find the _____ wire; it extends to 4 cm from the tip of the catheter.   thermistor

23. This thermodilution catheter can measure both _____ temperature and _____ output.   core
cardiac

24. You inject _____ ml of iced (or room temperature) _____ _____ into the _____ _____ port.   10   normal saline
right atrial

25. The cardiac output computer calculates the change in temperature from the _____ to the _____ port and then calculates the _____ _____.   proximal   distal
cardiac output

26. Systemic and pulmonary _____ _____ can be calculated using the formula on page 43 in *The Manual*. (Table 3.2 gives all the normals.)   vascular resistance

Review 25

Because these pressure readings are new to many of us, perhaps we need to review them again. Remember that normal varies for individuals and according to the accuracy of the measurements. See Figure 3–15 in *The Manual* for some of these answers.

1. CVP readings are measured by a (H₂O/Hg) manometer. H_2O

2. The normal CVP range is _____ to _____.   5   10 mm H_2O

3. CVP measures venous pressure in the _____ _____ _____ and reflects back pressure from the _____ _____.   superior vena cava
right atrium

4. Hemodynamic monitoring pressures are measured in mm (H₂O/Hg).   Hg

5. Mean right atrial pressures range from _____ mm Hg to _____ mm Hg.   2   6

6. The normal PAP is _____ systolic and _____ diastolic.   25   10

7. The (systolic/diastolic) pressure in the pulmonary artery is used to assess left ventricular function.   diastolic

8. Diastolic PAP above _____ may indicate that the left ventricle is not emptying completely.   12

9. PCWP is measured with the balloon _____.   inflated

10. PCWP of _____ to _____ is considered normal.   5   12

11. If the PCWP rises above _____, it may indicate that the left ventricle is not emptying completely.   12

Troubleshooting (pp. 43–47)
Review 26

1. The two most common problems are _____ of the wave form or a _____ problem.   damping
wedge

2. Wave forms are _____ if "something" is preventing the transmission of the blood wave.   damped

3. "Something" can include the catheter being _____ _____ _____ of the pulmonary artery.   against the wall

4. It may be possible to correct this by _____ the balloon and _____ the catheter a short distance.   inflating   floating

5. Other things causing damping may be _____ _____ in the tubing or transducer dome or _____ _____ on the distal tip of the catheter.

air bubbles
small clots

6. You can flush the system with several flushes of about _____ second each but avoid a long flush.

one

7. Why? _____
   _____
   _____

You may dislodge a blood clot and cause an embolus

8. If you cannot get a PCWP pressure, the _____ _____ _____ _____ may have floated backward out of place.

tip of the catheter

9. If you get a permanent PCWP pattern, the catheter may have migrated _____ and need to be repositioned.

forward

CLINICAL INFORMATION SYSTEMS (pp. 47–48)

Review 27

If you are fortunate enough to be in an ultramodern "computerized" CCU, then you need to familiarize yourself with your own system. If not, we will give you a brief description of what might be in your future.

1. Clinical information systems are also known as _____ _____ systems.

patient-data management

2. _____ at the bedside collect, process, and display patient care information.

Microcomputers

3. You may even progress to a completely _____ system.

paperless

4. To be most effective, the system needs to be integrated with _____, pharmacies, etc.

laboratories

5. It has been shown that computerized systems reduce the number of _____ errors but it has not been shown that _____ of care is improved.

charting
quality

Coronary Heart Disease

Review 1

1. Label the three coronary arteries in Figure 4.1.

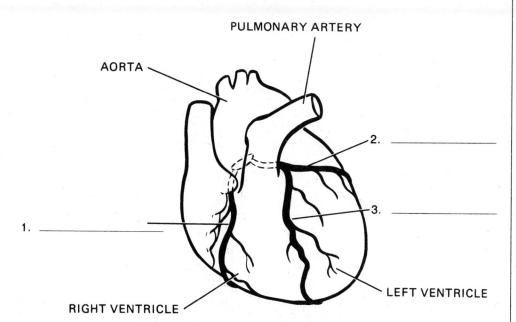

Figure 4.1. The coronary arteries of the heart.

1. right coronary artery
2. left circumflex artery
3. left anterior descending artery

THE CORONARY ARTERIES *(p. 49)*

An erroneous conception held by many patients (and perhaps a few nurses as well) is that the heart muscle feeds from the blood within its chambers. Actually, the myocardium (heart muscle) receives oxygen from blood carried by the coronary arteries. If a coronary arterial branch becomes blocked, the area of heart muscle it serves is deprived of oxygen. This can cause a heart attack. In order to understand heart attacks, you must have a basic knowledge of the coronary arteries.

Review 2

1. There are _____ *main* coronary arteries that carry blood to the myocardium.   **2**

2. These arteries leave the _____ just above the aortic valve.   **aorta**

3. These arteries are called the _____ coronary artery and the _____ coronary artery.   **left   right**

4. The left coronary artery divides into two large branches: the _____ _____ _____ _____ artery and the _____ _____ _____ artery.   **left anterior descending (LAD) left circumflex (LCA)**

Let's use abbreviations from now on.

5. The term *anterior* in LAD refers to the _____ part of the heart.   **front**

6. Thus, the LAD serves the anterior walls of _____ _____.   **both ventricles**

7. The LAD also supplies the anterior portion of the _____ _____.   **interventricular septum**

Stop and visualize this before continuing. Use Figure 4–1 in *The Manual.*

8. The other main branch of the left coronary artery is the _____ _____ _____ _____.   **left circumflex artery (LCA)**

9. This branch serves the left _____ and the _____ aspect of the left _____. (See Fig. 4–1 in *The Manual* if you are confused.)   **atrium   lateral ventricle**

10. The right coronary artery also arises from the _____.   **aorta**

11. It serves both the right _____ and the right _____.   **atrium   ventricle**

12. The right coronary artery comes down the (anterior/posterior) surface of the heart.   **posterior**

13. Thus it serves the _____ portion of the _____ ventricle.   **posterior   left**

14. It also serves the posterior portion of the _____ _____. (*Note:* Coronary artery patterns vary; this is the most common.)   **interventricular septum**

15. There (are/are not) many other small arterial branches that serve the myocardium.   **are**

16. The branches (do/do not) interconnect to form a network.   **do**

17. Each minute 250 mL of blood passes through the coronary arteries carrying oxygen to the myocardium.
    How many milliliters of blood per hour is this? _____   **15,000**
    How many liters per hour? _____   **15**
    How many milliliters of blood per 24 hours? _____   **360,000**
    How many liters of blood per 24 hours? _____   **360**
    (Imagine squeezing a bulb syringe about 70 times a minute and ejecting 15 liters of water into a sink for one hour. In effect, your heart does just that!)

CORONARY ATHEROSCLEROSIS (pp. 49–51)

Now you know a bit about the coronary arteries and the tremendous blood flow they handle constantly. Next let's think about the disease process that blocks them and interferes with the passage of this 360,000 mL of blood per day to the myocardium.

Review 3

1. The most common disease affecting the coronary arteries is _____.   **atherosclerosis**

2. Fatty substances (especially _____) form plaques on the inner lining of the blood vessels and narrow the passages.   **cholesterol**

3. Plaques tend to form at the _____ or _____ of the vessels.   **bifurcations   bends**

4. Plaques also may form where there is an _____ to vessel endothelium.   **injury**

5. Two of the cardiac risk factors that aggravate this process are _____ and _____.   **smoking hyperlipidemia**

6. _____ and _____ can accumulate on the plaques and release growth factors prompting _____ _____ cells to multiply.

7. These plaques can rupture and form a _____.

8. The critical determinant of CAD is (choose one or more):
   a. presence of atherosclerosis
   b. extent of arterial narrowing
   c. reduction in blood flow

9. The extent of arterial obstruction resulting in atherosclerosis is as follows:
   Grade ___ = _____% reduction of arterial lumen
   Grade ___ = _____% reduction of arterial lumen
   Grade ___ = _____% reduction of arterial lumen
   Grade ___ = _____% reduction of arterial lumen

10. Obstruction of less than _____% can usually be tolerated.

11. Grades _____ or _____ are considered significant obstructions.

12. Atherosclerosis is most dangerous when the narrowing involves the _____ main coronary artery.

13. This is because it would affect circulation through the left _____ _____ and the _____ arteries.

14. The left _____ _____ artery supplies blood to the anterior wall of the left and right ventricle.

Macrophages	platelets
smooth muscle	
thrombus	
b and c	
1	25
2	50
3	75
4	100
75	
3	4
left	
anterior descending	
circumflex	
anterior descending	

CAUSES OF CORONARY ATHEROSCLEROSIS (pp. 51–55)

To become more familiar with the dangers associated with risk factors, read some of the booklets published by the American Heart Association.* These pamphlets give you many of the facts you will need to answer the questions your patients may ask you about risk factors.

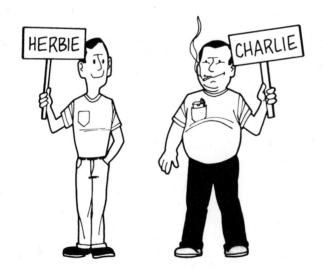

Figure 4.2

_____

* A.H.A. pamphlets: Controlling Your Risk Factors for Heart Attack, What's Your Risk of Heart Attack?, et al.

Review 4

Let's compare the risk of a heart attack to two middle-aged men. Good old Herbie is normal—and, I suspect, a little blah. He has none of the risk factors mentioned in *The Manual*. Chubbie Charlie, on the other hand, has a few problems. He is overweight, diabetic, has high blood pressure, and smokes two packs of cigarettes a day.

1. What would you guess are Charlie's chances of having a heart attack before the age of 65? 1 in _____. (Go ahead, guess.)

2, or a 50% chance

2. What about Herbie's? 1 in _____.

50, or a 2% chance

Furthermore, the American Heart Association warns people like Charlie that if they do have a heart attack, their chances of *dying* are much greater than Herbie's because Charlie is a *smoker.*

Review 5

Perhaps making profiles of individuals with low- and high-risk factors would help us visualize the *importance* of risk factors. The person with low-risk factors stands a lesser chance of developing CHD, while the person with many risk factors has a greater chance of developing CHD.

For each category listed, fill in the blanks in the following table. (Use numbers for blood pressure and serum cholesterol and short, descriptive terms for the other risk factors.) One pair is filled in as an example.

Table 4.1. Types of Risk Factors by Degree and Category

Categories	Lower Risk	Higher Risk
1. Sex	women	men
2. Sex and age		
3. Family history of CAD		
4. Metabolic diseases		
5. Weight		
6. Diet		
7. Serum cholesterol		
8. Triglycerides		
9. Blood pressure		
10. Cigarette smoking		
11. Activity		
12. Life-style		
13. Personality type		

Table 4.1. Answers

Categories	Lower Risk	Higher Risk
1. Sex	women	men
2. Sex and age	premenopausal women	men over 50
3. Family history of CAD	none	parent's MI before age 55
4. Metabolic diseases	none	especially diabetes, gout
5. Weight	normal	obese
6. Diet	low fat	high fat
7. Serum cholesterol	below 200	over 240
8. Triglycerides	below 200	above 200
9. Blood pressure	below 160/95	above 160/95
10. Cigarette smoking	nonsmoker	smoker
11. Activity	active	sedentary
12. Life-style	nonstressful	stressful
13. Personality type	type B	type A

LDL, VLDL, HDL, and CAD *(pp. 52–53)*

Review 6

From now on we will abbreviate coronary atherosclerotic disease as CAD. (Nurses don't mind abbreviations; it's the doctor's handwriting that we can't stand!) Lest mass confusion overcome us, let's spend a few minutes with all the initials used above.

1. Specifically, *The Manual* talks about two serum lipids, _____ and _____.

   cholesterol
   triglycerides

2. These two lipids are (soluble/insoluble) in plasma.

   insoluble

3. However, when combined with protein "carriers," they become _____, which are soluble.

   lipoproteins

4. There are three main classes of lipoprotein (initials, please). _____, _____, _____.

   LDL   VLDL
   HDL

5. One at a time now: VLDL stands for _____ _____ _____.

   very low-density lipoproteins

6. LDL stands for _____ _____.

   low-density lipoproteins

7. HDL stands for _____ _____.

   high-density lipoproteins

8. _____ carries more of the cholesterol in the blood.

   LDL

9. _____ carries more of the triglycerides in the blood.

   VLDL

10. Serum cholesterol and triglyceride levels (are/are not) necessarily related.

    are not

11. Now, let's oversimplify and classify these three as "good guys" or "bad guys." The "good guy" that seems to *protect* against CAD is _____.

    HDL

12. High levels of LDL (increase/decrease) the risk of CAD.

    increase

Remember the L stands for "lousy" in LDH and the H stands for "helpful." (It may help you remember which is which!)

THE CLINICAL SPECTRUM OF CORONARY ATHEROSCLEROSIS *(pp. 55–61)*

Review 7

To help you understand the full range of coronary atherosclerotic disease, complete the following:

1. CAD is caused by obstruction in the coronary _____.

   arteries

2. Minimal obstruction may not decrease the blood supply to the _____.

   myocardium

3. Minimal obstruction is unlikely to produce symptoms and may be discovered only after an _____.

   autopsy

4. Coronary arteries may be grossly obstructed but still not produce any _____.

   symptoms

5. This is because the oxygen needs of the myocardium have been supplied by _____ circulation.

   collateral

6. Coronary atherosclerosis (is/is not) synonymous with CAD.

   is not

7. Inadequate blood supply to the myocardium results in a lack of _____ for the cardiac cells.

   oxygen

8. Insufficient oxygenation is called _____.

   ischemia

9. Myocardial ischemia causes chest pain known as _____ _____.

   angina pectoris

10. In order of severity, the three clinical patterns of CAD are *stable angina pectoris*, _____ _____, and _____ _____ _____.

    unstable angina
    acute myocardial infarction

Angina Pectoris (pp. 55–56)

Angina pectoris is one of the most important symptoms of CAD. Note how carefully the chest pain is described in *The Manual*. Because you will have to decide whether a patient is experiencing angina, you will need a clear understanding of the clinical picture.

Review 8

1. Angina is characterized by its _____ (or precordial) location.

2. It frequently radiates to any of several sites, including the arms, _____, _____, _____, and _____ _____.

3. The pain (is/is not) relieved by changes in breathing or position.

4. The pain is usually described as a _____ or a _____.

5. The pain often begins during _____ _____.

6. It usually _____ as soon as activity ceases.

7. Thus, it is termed _____ of _____.

8. It is possible for _____ as well as physical stress to induce angina.

9. Any stress that increases the heart _____ or blood _____ may induce angina.

10. Angina generally lasts _____ to _____ minutes.

11. It is almost always relieved by _____.

12. Nitroglycerin _____ the coronary arteries and _____ capacitance vessels.

13. This (increases/decreases) the blood and oxygen supply to the myocardium.

14. The most common side effect of nitroglycerin is _____.

15. If nitroglycerin does not relieve pain, you should suspect the pain (is/is not) due to angina of effort.

substernal
neck
jaw   shoulders   upper back
is not
pressure   tightness
physical exertion
stops
angina   effort
emotional
rate   pressure
1   5
nitroglycerin
dilates   venous
increases
headache
is not

Diagnosis of Angina Pectoris (pp. 56–57)
Review 9

1. In diagnosis of angina pectoris the most important thing is _____ _____.

2. If you are questioning a patient about a chest pain episode, there are four areas of importance: _____ _____, _____ _____, _____ _____, and _____ _____ _____.

3. Stress tests may be used to induce ECG evidence of myocardial _____. (If you haven't observed one, make arrangements to do so.)

4. Chest pain during a stress test (is/is not) defined as a positive result.

5. Positive stress tests require _____ _____.

6. One of the nuclear scanning techniques used in diagnosis of CAD is _____ _____.

7. During exercise testing, ventricular muscle areas with reduced blood flow contract (normally/abnormally).

8. An IV injection of a _____ _____ is given during the peak exercise period.

9. The nuclear camera will record abnormal ventricular contractions in _____ areas.

10. The most definitive method of diagnosis is _____ _____.

11. This involves inserting a catheter through a peripheral artery into the root of the _____ and injecting radiopaque dye into the _____ _____ _____.

patient's history
location (central)   duration (brief)   quality (oppressive) relation to effort
ischemia
is not
ECG changes
radionuclide angiography
abnormally
radioactive isotope
ischemic
coronary arteriography
aorta   two coronary arteries

12. List three things coronary arteriography can show: _____ _____ _____
    _____, _____ _____ _____, and _____ _____
    _____ _____.

13. Two other diagnostic studies are _____ _____ and
    _____.

14. In cardiac catheterization, catheters are run into the heart _____ and the
    great _____.

15. Measurements are then made of the _____ and _____
    _____ in these areas.

16. In ventriculography, a radiopaque dye is inserted through a catheter placed in the
    _____ _____.

17. The "motion pictures" resulting are (more/less) precise than radionuclide pictures.

number of vessels involved
extent of involvement
degree of collateral circulation

cardiac catheterization
ventriculography

chambers
vessels

pressures
oxygen concentrations

left ventricle

more

Stable and Variant Angina Pectoris (pp. 57–58)

I'll bet you knew that angina pectoris couldn't be so "stable" and simple. You were right! For years doctors have been plagued by patients with "variant" symptoms: patients who refused to conform to nice, clinical patterns of angina, yet who obviously had sick hearts. So now we have a classification for them: variant angina pectoris.

Review 10

To refine your knowledge about stable and variant angina, place an S (stable) or a V (variant) in front of the most appropriate statements below.

____ 1. No pain or ECG evidence during exercise testing

____ 2. Fixed narrowing of arteries

____ 3. Also known as "classic" angina

____ 4. May be relieved by calcium antagonists

____ 5. Effectively relieved by calcium antagonists

____ 6. Relieved by rest

____ 7. Caused by coronary artery spasm

____ 8. Relieved with nitroglycerin

____ 9. Pain at rest

____ 10. Cyclic pain pattern

____ 11. Induced by physical activity

____ 12. Induced by emotional stress

____ 13. Also known as Prinzmetal's angina

____ 14. Often 75% narrowing of 2 or 3 arteries

1. V
2. S
3. S
4. S
5. V
6. S
7. V
8. S
9. V
10. V
11. S
12. S
13. V
14. S

Unstable Angina (p. 58)

As you now realize, angina pectoris is only a symptom of CAD. It is a warning that the heart isn't getting all the blood it needs at that moment. Changes in the circulatory condition and patterns of the syndrome result in a progression of severity: stable or variant; then unstable; and finally the most ominous, acute myocardial infarction. Picture this progression by using your imagination. You could relate the patterns to horses: "stable," predictable ones or the "variantly" behaving, confusing ones; then the "unstable," more dangerous ones; and finally, the "acute" situation, the rider unseated, writhing on the ground. Form your own pictures to remember these terms because you are about ready to meet more new terms. (Just don't confuse "variant" and "unstable.")

Review 11

1. Unstable angina ranks in severity between _____ _____ and _____ _____ _____.

   stable angina   acute myocardial infarction

2. A common feature of unstable angina is clinical (stability/instability).

   instability

3. Unstable angina pain usually lasts (1 to 5/5 to 10/10 to 20) minutes.

   10 to 20

4. Over time the pattern of unstable angina occurs _____ _____, can be induced by (less/greater) exertion, and (often/seldom) occurs at rest.

   more frequently   less   often

5. Nitroglycerin's effect on unstable angina is _____ _____ _____.

   incomplete or none

6. ECG commonly shows signs of _____.

   ischemia

7. ECG (does/does not) show signs of acute myocardial infarction.

   does not

8. Unstable angina is (more/less) severe than stable angina.

   more

9. The immediate forerunner of acute myocardial infarction is _____ _____.

   unstable   angina

Acute Myocardial Infarction *(pp. 58–61)*

Review 12

Now let's use your knowledge of the coronary arterial anatomy to see what happens in acute myocardial infarction.

1. As you know, insufficient oxygenation of tissues is called _____.

   ischemia

2. If ischemia is severe or prolonged, tissue _____ may occur.

   destruction

3. This is called _____.

   necrosis

4. Necrotic muscle is also called _____ muscle.

   infarcted

5. A myocardial infarction means a local area of heart muscle is _____ or _____.

   dead   infarcted

6. What your patient calls a heart attack, you call a _____ _____.

   myocardial infarction

7. You usually abbreviate that to _____ or _____.

   MI   AMI

8. Nearly all AMIs are due to _____ _____.

   coronary atherosclerosis

9. The event producing an acute MI may be called a coronary _____ or coronary _____.

   thrombosis occlusion

10. In actual practice, the terms *myocardial infarction, heart attack,* and *coronary* are used interchangeably. (True/False)

    True

11. A coronary artery may be blocked if a _____ develops on the rough atherosclerotic plaques.

    clot

12. A coronary artery may be blocked if bleeding occurs under the plaques. That's called _____ _____.

    subintimal hemorrhage

13. Or a piece of plaque may _____ _____ and swim away to block a small artery.

    break off

14. Autopsies have shown AMIs (can/cannot) occur without clots or complete arterial obstruction.

    can

15. Two possible explanations for Question 14 are: _____ _____ _____ _____ _____ _____.

    Sudden intense oxygen demand (due to exercise or stress) that the arteries can't supply or coronary arterial spasm complicating an existing coronary artery disease.

16. Blockage of the (right/left) coronary artery is usually more serious.

    left

17. The left coronary artery divides into two main branches, the _____ and the _____. | LAD   LCA

18. They primarily serve the (anterior/posterior) portion of the left heart. | anterior

19. Thus, occlusion of the left coronary artery is likely to cause (anterior/posterior) MI. | anterior

20. The right coronary artery travels down the back of the heart and supplies the (inferior/superior) portion of the left ventricle. | inferior

21. The inferior part of the heart is also called the _____ portion. | diaphragmatic

22. Occlusion of the right coronary artery is likely to cause an _____ _____ MI. | inferior (or diaphragmatic)

23. If an infarction involves the anterior wall of the left ventricle and the anterior portion of the interventricular septum, the infarction would be termed an _____ MI. | anteroseptal

24. In this case, the occluded coronary artery is the _____. | LAD

25. An infarction involving the anterior and lateral aspects of the left ventricle would be termed an _____ MI. | anterolateral

26. An infarction involving the inferior and lateral walls of the left ventricle is termed an _____ MI. | inferiolateral

27. An infarction of only the right ventricle (is/is not) rare. | is

28. A right ventricular infarction may occur with an _____ myocardial infarction. | inferior

29. This is because the right coronary artery supplies both the right ventricle and the _____ wall of the _____ _____. | inferior   left ventricle

30. The extent of an infarction depends on the _____ of the artery obstructed and the degree of _____ _____ available. | size   collateral circulation

31. If an area of infarction extends clear through the ventricular wall, it is a _____ MI. | transmural

32. An infarction that does not extend through the full thickness of the ventricular wall is termed nontransmural, _____, or _____. | intramural   subendocardial

Now let's update those terms.

33. A more modern way to categorize MIs is by the changes in the _____ wave of the ECG. | Q

34. Look back at Figure 3.4. The Q wave is part of the _____ complex which shows ventricular _____. | QRS   depolarization

35. A Q-wave infarction used to be called a _____ infarction and is medium to _____ in size. | transmural   large

36. A non-Q-wave infarction may (or may not) extend from the _____ to the _____ wall. | subendocardial   epicardial

37. While the hospital mortality rate is _____ for Q wave infarctions, the two-year mortality rate is the same for Q-wave and non–Q-wave infarctions. | greater

38. If Mr. Kardiak has a non-Q-wave infarction you will be especially alert about _____ _____ after the initial infarction for a possible extension of his MI. | 10 days

39. You will probably see more (Q wave/non–Q-wave) infarctions in your CCU. | Q wave

Review 13

Label Zones I, II, and III on the infarcted area in Figure 4.3.

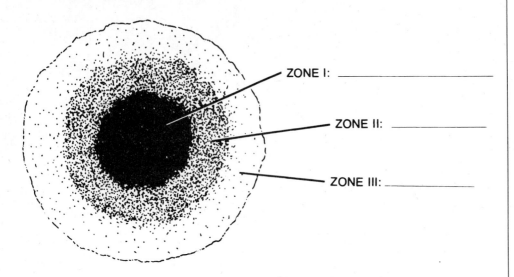

ZONE I: _____

ZONE II: _____

ZONE III: _____

Zone I: Infarction

Zone II: Injury

Zone III: Ischemia

Figure 4.3. Three zones of tissue damage associated with acute myocardial infarction.

1. Zone I is (temporarily/permanently) damaged.

2. Zone II may recover if adequate _____ is restored.

3. Zone III (often/rarely) recovers.

4. Zones II and III are not distinct and together are called the _____ zone.

permanently

circulation

often

border

Review 14

You have learned so much in this chapter. Suppose we introduce three patients to make this seem more real. Come on in and join the gang at Myoville General Hospital. Meet our rather colorful patients and see if you can visualize what has happened to their coronary arteries. Use Figure 4.4 to help you.

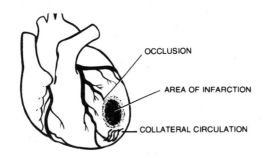

Figure 4.4A

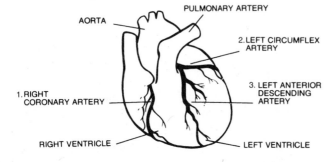

Figure 4.4B

Patient 1: Mr. T. Brown

Draw a blood clot obstructing the coronary artery where the line for artery 1 touches the artery on Figure 4.4B. Coronary arteriography demonstrates an obstruction at this point.

1. From the coronary arteriographic findings, you conclude that the _____ _____ ar-tery is obstructed.

   right coronary

2. This means that the _____ _____ and _____ _____ may be deprived of an adequate blood supply.

   right atrium   right ventricle

3. Far more important, obstruction of the right coronary artery affects the inferior section of the _____ _____.

   left ventricle

4. It also affects the posterior portion of the _____ septum.

   interventricular

5. The obstruction of Mr. Brown's right coronary artery involves mainly the (superior/inferior) portion of his heart.

   inferior

6. The inferior portion of the heart lies near what anatomical landmark? _____

   diaphragm

7. Therefore, the ECG diagnosis of Mr. Brown's infarction will be classified as _____ or _____.

   inferior   diaphragmatic

Patient 2: Mr. Forrest Green

Draw an obstruction of the coronary artery where the line for artery 2 touches the artery on Figure 4.4B.

1. Mr. Green's coronary arteriogram shows that the _____ _____ artery is obstructed.

   left circumflex

2. This artery provides blood to the left _____ and the lateral aspect of the left _____.

   atrium
   ventricle

3. Mr. Green's ECG reveals changes in the _____ wall of the left ventricle.

   lateral

Patient 3: Mrs. Misty Blue

Draw a plaque obstructing the coronary artery where the line for artery 3 meets the artery on Figure 4.4B.

1. Mrs. Blue's coronary arteriogram shows that the _____ _____ _____ artery is obstructed.

   left anterior
   descending

2. This artery services the (anterior/posterior) wall of the _____ _____.

   anterior   left ventricle

3. It also serves the (anterior/posterior) portion of the _____ septum.

   anterior   interventricular

4. If Mrs. Blue's infarction involves the anterior portion of the left ventricle and the interventricular septum, it is termed an _____.

   anteroseptal

5. An obstruction of the left coronary artery *before* its bifurcation would deprive the (anterior/posterior) portion of the _____ _____, the anterior portion of the _____ _____, and also the _____ aspect of the left ventricle.

   anterior   left ventricle
   interventricular septum   lateral

6. This could cause an extensive _____ MI.

   anterior

7. Read some of the ECGs of patients with MI. How many of these diagnostic terms can you find? _____ _____

   Probably all

8. Doesn't it make you feel good to know what they mean?

   I hope so!

Now let's try a few review questions on coronary heart disease. By the time you finish these, you should have a much better understanding of this subject than you did when you started!

TERMINOLOGY REVIEW—QUESTIONS

Review 15

You may have learned some new terms or relearned some old ones in this chapter. Test yourself by placing the definitions numbers in front of the correct terms.

Definitions	*Terms*
1. provide blood to nourish the heart muscle	_____angina pectoris
2. muscle layer of the heart	_____atherosclerosis
3. narrowing of arteries due to fatty deposits	_____collateral circulation
4. inner lining of arteries	_____coronary arteries
5. occurs when blood supply to myocardium is insufficient	_____intima
6. secondary blood supply	_____myocardium

1. chest pain due to ischemia	_____unstable angina
2. longer lasting, more serious angina	_____plaque
3. follows classic, established pattern	_____variant angina
4. pain from coronary artery spasm	_____stable angina
5. fatty deposits	_____subintimal
6. underneath the lining of an artery	_____angina pectoris
7. resulting from lack of oxygen	_____necrosis
8. local death of cells	_____ischemia

1. irreversible myocardial damage	_____anterolateral infarction
2. area of injury and ischemia	_____border zone
3. involves anterior wall of left ventricle	_____infarction
4. involves diaphragmatic wall of left ventricle	_____Q-wave infarction
5. involves anterior and lateral walls	_____anterior infarction
6. involves anterior wall of left ventricle and interventricular septum	_____inferior infarction
7. larger myocardial infarction	_____non–Q-wave infarction
8. shows nonspecific ECG changes	_____anteroseptal infarction

Turn the page to check your answers.

TERMINOLOGY REVIEW—ANSWERS

Definitions	*Answers*	*Terms*

1. provide blood to nourish the heart muscle	5	angina pectoris
2. muscle layer of the heart	3	atherosclerosis
3. narrowing of arteries due to fatty deposits	6	collateral circulation
4. inner lining of arteries	1	coronary arteries
5. occurs when blood supply to myocardium is insufficient	4	intima
6. secondary blood supply	2	myocardium

1. chest pain due to ischemia	2	unstable angina
2. longer lasting, more serious angina	5	plaque
3. follows classic, established pattern	4	variant angina
4. pain from coronary artery spasm	3	stable angina
5. fatty deposits	6	subintimal
6. underneath the lining of an artery	1	angina pectoris
7. resulting from lack of oxygen	8	necrosis
8. local death of cells	7	ischemia

1. irreversible myocardial damage	5	anterolateral infarction
2. area of injury and ischemia	2	border zone
3. involves anterior wall of left ventricle	1	infarction
4. involves diaphragmatic wall of left ventricle	7	Q-wave infarction
5. involves anterior and lateral walls	3	anterior infarction
6. involves anterior wall of left ventricle and interventricular septum	4	inferior infarction
7. larger myocardial infarction	8	non–Q-wave infarction
8. shows nonspecific ECG changes	6	anteroseptal infarction

5

Acute Myocardial Infarction

THE ONSET OF THE ATTACK *(p. 63)*

Table 5.1 (*The Manual,* p. 64) is so important! You need to know those symptoms. Learn them by writing out the five headings and then from memory replicate the signs and symptoms as listed. Then let's go to the ER at Myoville General.

Review 1

Mr. A is brought to the Emergency Room at 3 A.M. He is gray-faced, obviously in pain, and gasping for breath.

Nurse: What seems to be the problem?
Mr. A: This pain—I woke up with it. I feel like I'm gonna die.
Nurse: Can you tell me what the pain feels like?
Mr. A: Like a truck sitting on my chest.
Nurse: Exactly where does it hurt?
Mr. A: (*Strikes midchest with clenched fist.*) Here and all across. It's strange; my left elbow hurts, and my jaw, too.
Nurse: Has the pain eased up any since it began?
Mr. A: No it just won't go away. I tried Alka-Seltzer and then a little whiskey—nothing helps.
Nurse: When the pain began, did you sweat?
Mr. A: My pajamas were soaked.
Nurse: Were you sick at your stomach?
Mr. A: Was I? I vomited twice already. I knew I shouldn't have eaten both lasagna and spaghetti last night.
Nurse: When did you get short of breath?
Mr. A: Right after the pain began. I couldn't get my breath.

Mrs. B comes to the Emergency Room an hour later. She is doubled up with pain, white-faced, dyspneic, and obviously frightened.

Nurse: You seem to be in pain.
Mrs. B: Oh, my chest . . .

Nurse: What is the pain like?

Mrs. B: It's like a knife—a sharp pain—it stabs here (*indicates left side of chest with one finger*).

Nurse: Is the pain continuous?

Mrs. B: No. It comes and goes.

Nurse: How about breathing?

Mrs. B: I don't dare take a deep breath; it makes the pain worse.

Nurse: Did the pain start all at once?

Mrs. B: It began gradually, but it's gotten worse.

Nurse: Have you vomited or been nauseated?

Mrs. B: I keep belching all the time. Have I had a heart attack?

Review 2

Let's analyze the history and symptoms of these patients by means of a series of questions. Then read the discussion that follows.

1. Is there good reason to suspect from the history that Mr. A has had a myocardial infarction? (Yes/No) _____

Yes, the symptoms Mr. A. describes should certainly make you suspect an acute myocardial infarction.

2. What about Mrs. B? (Yes/No) _____

No, Mrs. B.'s history is not suggestive of myocardial infarction.

3. What is the most important symptom in Mr. A.'s history to suggest acute myocardial infarction? _____

The most important symptom is severe substernal pain which persists. This symptom alone should make you suspicious. Be aware that people interpret "pain" differently. I'm reminded of a lady who insisted, "I had absolutely no pain with my heart attack. It just felt like an elephant was sitting on my chest." Now, to me, that's pain.

4. What other symptoms of his further this suspicion? _____

Pain to elbow and jaw, sweating, nausea and vomiting, shortness of breath.

5. Is the localized, knifelike pain Mrs. B. experienced characteristic of acute myocardial infarction? (Yes/No) _____

No

6. What about the relationship of Mrs. B.'s chest pain to breathing? Is this a common story? (Yes/No) _____

No, pain on breathing isn't a common complaint with AMI.

60

7. How important do you think it is for a nurse to be able to recognize acute myocardial infarction? (Very/Not very) _____

_____

_____

_____

8. There are six cardinal symptoms of an acute MI. By now you should know them. They are _____ _____, _____, _____, _____, _____, _____ _____.

9. Is the pain always in the chest? _____

10. Other likely sites for MI pain are _____, _____, or _____.

11. And just to complicate matters, when an MI shows up on an ECG and the patient denies any symptoms, it is called a _____ MI.

Very important. Your ability to recognize the symptoms of an MI, whether in a postoperative or emergency room patient, or in your friends or family, may save a life.

substernal pain   sweating
nausea   vomiting   dyspnea
sudden weakness

no

arms   neck   shoulders

silent

CHANGES IN THE HEART *(pp. 63–64)*

Review 3

Now, start with the atherosclerotic process and put in order the changes that occur in a typical uncomplicated MI.

Scrambled

a. atherosclerosis
b. cellular necrosis begins in 20 to 40 minutes
c. area blood flow interrupted
d. removal of necrotic tissue in 4 to 7 days
e. myocardial necrosis in 8 to 12 hours
f. myocardial cells in area stop contracting within 1 minute
g. plaque ruptures
h. leukocytes infiltrate
i. thrombus forms
j. subendocardial through to epicardial necrosis
k. area of myocardium becomes cyanotic
l. scar formation begins in 2 to 3 weeks
m. plaque forms
n. scar formation complete in 2 months

In Order of Occurrence

a
m
g
i
c
k
f
b
j
e
h
d
l
n

Review 4

Now a few more questions on these important "changes."

1. first surface to become ischemic: _____

2. necrosis spreads from subendocardial to _____

3. necrosis spreads from myocardium to _____

4. most at risk for necrosis: _____

5. last surface area to reperfuse: _____

subendocardial

myocardial

epicardium

subendocardium

subendocardial

Review 5

To fix in your mind the sequence of these events (without looking back at the "Scrambler"), match "Changes and Times."

Changes	Times	Answers
a. myocardial necrosis	_____ 1 min	c
b. scar formation begins	_____ 20 to 40 min	f
c. cellular contraction stops	_____ 8 to 12 hrs	a
d. removal of necrotic tissue	_____ 4 to 7 days	d
e. scar formation complete	_____ 2 to 3 wks	b
f. necrosis starts at subendocardial surface	_____ 2 months	e

To further reinforce this, write out the sequence of "Changes" in the order they happen.

THE CLINICAL COURSE IMMEDIATELY AFTER INFARCTION (pp. 64–65)

Review 6

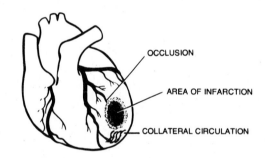

Figure 5.1A

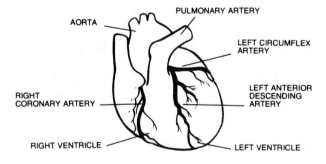

Figure 5.1B

Figure 5.1A shows an MI with collateral circulation. Use Figure 5.1B and draw a small-sized infarction with good collateral circulation.

1. Let's say this heart continues to pump normally and the rate and rhythm remain normal. You would expect this patient on admission to be in (no/great) distress.

   no

2. Now draw a larger infarction with very little collateral circulation. This may _____ the heart's pumping action or disturb the heart's _____ and _____.

   decrease   rate   rhythm

Review 7

3. Do all patients with acute MI develop complications? (Yes/No) — No

4. Can you be certain that a patient with a small infarction won't develop complications? (Yes/No) — No

5. If a patient has a large infarction, can you be certain that complications will develop? (Yes/No) — No

6. In other words, complications can develop in _____ patient at _____ time! — any   any (*never forget this*)

7. Without sufficient oxygen your heart won't pump effectively. So decreased oxygenation leads to decreased _____. — pumping

8. Decreased pumping can lead to _____ _____. — heart failure

9. When the left ventricle is severely injured and can't pump out enough blood to meet the body's needs, vital organs such as the _____ and _____ are deprived of adequate blood and oxygen. — brain   kidneys

10. As a result, the blood pressure _____. — falls

11. Urinary output _____. — decreases

12. The skin becomes _____ and _____. — cold   clammy

13. The failing heart struggles to compensate, so it pumps _____. — faster

14. The pulse rate (increases/decreases). — increases

15. Questions 7 through 12 describe what condition? _____ _____. — cardiogenic shock

16. Impaired oxygenation can also upset the _____ and _____ of the heartbeat. — rate   rhythm

17. This produces _____. — arrhythmias

18. Arrhythmias can cause _____ death. — sudden

19. Arrhythmias can occur at _____ time in _____ patient. — any   any

20. The most common lethal arrhythmia is _____ _____. — ventricular fibrillation

21. In ventricular fibrillation the heart muscle _____ and (does/does not) pump. (That's enough for now, you will learn much more about this later.) — quivers   does not

THE DIAGNOSIS OF ACUTE MYOCARDIAL INFARCTION *(p. 65)*

Review 8

Mr. Kardiak is rushed into the ER at 2 A.M. There are three steps (possibly four) that are necessary to make a definitive diagnosis of AMI (acute myocardial infarction).

First Step

1. Probably most important is the _____ _____. — patient's history

2. So you won't ever forget them, the six symptoms that you look for are: _____ _____ _____, _____ _____ _____, _____, _____ _____. — severe substernal pain, nausea and vomiting, dyspnea, sudden weakness

Second Step

3. To make a definitive diagnosis, you must have positive _____ changes. — ECG

4. The initial ECG will (always/not always) show AMI changes. — not always

5. In an MI, serial ECGs (will/will not) show characteristic changes and (will/will not) show the actual extent of damage. — will   will not

63

6. ECG changes may be equivocal (on admision), then _____ _____ are important.	lab studies
7. When muscle cells are injured they release _____.	enzymes
8. Three enzymes we are especially interested in are __, ____, and ___ (initials, please!).	CK SGOT LDH

Enzyme Studies (p. 65)

To remember the order in which the enzymes rise, drop the S off SGOT (it stands for serum anyway) and then put the enzymes in alphabetical order. CK, GOT, LDH. Watching these lab reports on your cardiac patients is fascinating. Sometimes the enzymes reach frighteningly high levels (which usually means extensive myocardial damage), and then you wish you could pack your patient's heart in cotton balls to protect it.

CK—The Early Bird
Review 9

1. CK is released after damage to the heart muscle, _____ muscles, or _____ _____.	skeletal the brain
2. Thus, CK elevations may occur after an MI, or a fracture with _____ injury, or a _____ with brain damage.	muscle stroke
3. _____ medication given to a patient may cause a slight elevation of CK.	Intramuscular (IM)
4. An isoenzyme of CK specific for myocardial necrosis is called _____.	CK–MB
5. CK rises almost immediately, within _____ to _____ hours after an MI.	2 6
6. It usually peaks within _____ hours.	24
7. Thus, it makes sense to measure CK levels on admission, _____ _____ later, and at the end of day _____ and _____.	24 hours 2 3
8. CK–MB is "quicker on the draw." It begins to rise _____ to _____ hours after the AMI, peaks at _____ hours, and may return to normal in _____ hours.	2 3 12 24
9. CK–MB greater than ____% of the total CK is almost certainly diagnostic of an AMI.	5
11. Mr. Kardiak probably has an extensive AMI if CK–MB elevates _____ and _____ _____ than usual.	immediately remains longer

SGOT—The Second Riser
Review 10

1. Now to throw off our alphabetical progression, you can add three letters to the SGOT and it is called _____. (Sounds like a sugar-free sweetener, doesn't it?)	AST/SGOT
1. While CK usually elevates within 2 to 6 hours after an MI, it takes SGOT about _____ hours to begin rising.	8
2. CK peaks in 24 hours; SGOT peaks between _____ and _____ hours.	24 48
3. SGOT usually returns to normal after _____ to _____ days.	4 6
4. SGOT also increases in noncardiac-related diseases, particularly _____ disease.	liver

LDH—The Slowpoke
Review 11

1. LDH doesn't usually peak until the _____ or _____ day after an MI.	3rd 4th
2. LDH usually returns to normal about the _____ or _____ day after an MI.	6th 7th

3. Lab tests for LDH would be done on the _____, _____, and _____ days if the diagnosis is unconfirmed. | 3rd 4th 5th

4. LDH elevations also occur in _____, _____, and _____ _____ diseases. | pulmonary renal skeletal muscle

5. If the ratio of the 2 LDH isoenzymes, LDH1/LDH2, is greater than _____, it indicates myocardial necrosis. | 1.0

6. Now to set things straight (or confuse you totally): a diagnosis of AMI (can/cannot) be made solely on elevated enzyme levels but negative enzyme studies (do/do not) rule out an AMI. (How about a cup of coffee?) | cannot do not

Radionuclide Imaging *(pp. 67–68)*

Review 12

1. If other diagnostic evidence is missing or misleading, radionuclide imaging (can/cannot) be used to help diagnose an MI. | can

2. Two basic forms of radionuclide imaging are "_____-spot" and "_____-spot" imaging. | hot   cold

3. "Hot-spot" imaging uses IV _____ 99^m pyrophosphate. | technetium

4. Necrotic myocardium shows a (greater/lesser) uptake of the IV technetium. | greater

5. This increased radioactivity is called a "_____ _____." | "hot spot"

6. "Hot-spot" imaging is more reliable for (transmural/nontransmural) infarctions. | transmural

7. "Cold-spot" imaging uses _____-201. | thallium

8. Necrotic myocardium shows (no/a greater) uptake of thallium-201. | no

9. Thus, a void or "(cold/hot) spot" shows the area of necrosis. | cold

10. A new infarct (can/cannot) be differentiated from an old infarct with thallium. | cannot

11. Thallium can be used with _____ _____ to help diagnose the ischemia of angina and unstable angina. | exercise testing

Cardiac Radiography *(pp. 68–69)*

Review 13

1. Chest x-rays will show the _____ of the heart chambers and status of the _____ system. | size pulmonary

2. If Mr. Kardiak's condition allows, x-ray views taken will be both _____ and _____. | frontal lateral

3. Which frontal view is best, PA or AP? _____ | PA

4. The _____ view tends to _____ the size of the heart's chambers. | AP   exaggerate

5. Diagnosis of an enlarged heart is called _____. | cardiomegaly

6. The normal heart (frontal view) should occupy _____% or less of the total thoracic width. | 50

7. _____ ratio is the term for this relationship. | Cardio/thoracic

8. Larger ratios are found in patients with _____ _____, _____ _____, _____ _____, and some _____ diseases. | heart failure   valvular lesions intracardiac shunts pulmonary

9. Pulmonary _____, caused by _____ heart failure, can be seen on x-ray. | congestion   left

65

THE ACUTE PHASE OF MYOCARDIAL INFARCTION (p. 69)

Review 14

Let's recap. The doctor has admitted the patient to the CCU because of suspected myocardial infarction. The history, ECG, and enzymes all say MI. What can you expect now? Suppose we take a look at three patients who illustrate the "three broad patterns" described in *The Manual*.

1. Mrs. Glutton is a collage of risk factors. But after her pain subsides, she becomes a pain; she complains loudly about the CCU diet (low cholesterol, low calorie, low sodium), she's dying for a cigarette, she misses her favorite TV soap opera. Thankfully, she recovers uneventfully and goes home. Lucky? Or just a small infarct with good collateral circulation?

2. Mr. Thirty-nine is so young. No one can really believe he has had an MI, not even with all the diagnostic evidence that exists. He has had occasional arrhythmias, but he seems to be doing so well you just can't take them seriously. You are chatting with him one afternoon with your back to the monitor, and he is telling you a joke—but he never makes it to the punch line. Ventricular fibrillation stops him. Does he die? What do you think?

3. Mr. Hectic is so cold and clammy on admission that you wonder if he came by refrigerated van rather than by ambulance. You breathe a prayer and stick an IV needle into a vein that is hardly even there. From then on you fight; the next day, you are almost certain Mr. Hectic won't be there. And you are right.

Remember these are only general patterns of the course after an MI. Next time, Mrs. Glutton may be a number 3, and the young, strong thirty-niner may be a number 1. But don't count on it.

1. The most characteristic aspect of the acute phase is _____.

   unpredictability

2. Mrs. Glutton develops no complications so she will probably leave the CCU in _____ to _____ days.

   2   3

3. CCUs were developed (primarily) to treat _____ _____ _____ (and he could be any age and probably is older).

   Mr. Thirty Nine

4. There is about a _____% likelihood that Mr. Hectic will die. (If your good care saves him, it's a real accomplishment.)

   70

THE COMPLICATIONS OF ACUTE MYOCARDIAL INFARCTION (pp. 69–75)

Review 15

1. Your first objective as a CCU nurse is to _____ _____.

   prevent complications

2. You will see plenty of arrhythmias since _____% of AMIs develop them.

   90

3. Arrhythmias are dangerous because they reduce the heart's ability to _____.

   pump

4. This can lead to acute _____ _____.

   heart failure

5. The biggest danger is _____ _____; it can occur at _____ _____.

   sudden death   any time

6. In addition to disturbances in rate and _____, you watch Mr Kardiak's monitor for _____ _____.

   rhythm
   conduction blocks

7. Two general causes of conduction blocks are _____ (or necrosis) of _____ pathways and increased _____ _____.

   ischemia   conduction
   vagal activity

Heart Failure (pp. 70–71)
Review 16

1. You will probably see some signs of heart failure in about _____% of your patients.

   60

2. Usually, heart failure results when the _____ of the heart is reduced due to the _____ and _____.

   contractility
   infarction necrosis

3. A second cause of heart failure is _____ or infarction of the _____ muscles impairing the effectiveness of the valve leaflets.

   rupture   papillary

4. If papillary muscles rupture and _____ fail, blood backs up into the _____ _____ during systole.

   valves   left atrium

5. The _____ _____ filling pressure increases and leads to heart failure.

   left ventricular

6. A third cause of heart failure is rupture of the ventricular _____.

   septum

7. Then blood flows from the higher pressured _____ ventricle into the _____ ventricle and overloads the _____ ventricle.

   left   right
   right

8. Blood remains in the _____ capillaries and the increased volumes lead to _____ heart failure.

   pulmonary
   right

9. If you discover a new, loud _____ murmur, you would suspect an _____ _____.

   systolic
   interventricular rupture

10. This could be confirmed if the pulmonary artery catheter shows a marked increase in _____ saturation in the (right/left) heart.

    oxygen   right

11. The most severe form of heart failure is _____ _____.

    cardiogenic shock

12. Then the heart fails to provide adequate _____ to vital _____ and tissues.

    oxygen   organs

13. The mortality in cardiogenic shock patients is about _____%.

    70

Thromboembolism (p. 71)

Before we begin our discussion of thromboembolism, we must clarify a basic point. A *thrombus* is a clot sitting around the home fires. When a thrombus turns tramp, it becomes an embolus. An *embolus* roams through the circulatory system "just looking for a home."

If you are still confused, here is one more hint. You have seen the term *thromboembolism,* but have you ever seen *embothrombolism?* No, the thrombus comes first; it becomes an embolus only when it moves.

Review 17

1. After an MI, there seems to be an increased incidence of clots, or _____.

   thrombi

2. The thrombi forming in the deep veins of the legs are called _____ thrombi.

   peripheral

3. Thrombi forming inside the heart's chambers are called _____ thrombi.

   mural

5. The infarcted myocardium may contract poorly and this leads to _____ and _____ which increase thrombus formation.

   stasis
   turbulence

6. You are more likely to see mural thrombi in an (inferior/anterior) AMI, especially if the left ventricular _____ is infarcted.

   anterior
   apex

7. Emboli are classified according to (where they originate/where they eventually lodge).

   where they eventually lodge

8. The three classifications of emboli are _____, _____, and _____.

   pulmonary   cerebral
   peripheral

Pulmonary Embolism (p. 71)
First, let's discuss emboli that lodge in the lungs. A large clot blocking off a major artery in the lungs produces unforgettable symptoms. Your patient is suddenly frantic for

breath, shocky, apprehensive, and in terrible pain. Not all pulmonary emboli block off major arteries, so sometimes the picture is less grim.

I would like to let a nurse friend of mine, Joan, tell what it's like to have a pulmonary emboli. Although her embolism wasn't caused by MI, the symptoms were the same. Joan says, "I had just had a complete physical, and as I trotted out of the doctor's office, I was stabbed with a knifelike pain in my right chest. I know exactly what a patient means when he says, 'the pain took my breath away.' But I didn't dare return to the doctor's office; I could just see the 'hypochondriac' label floating there." So Joan rationalized, "Must have pulled a muscle opening that door." By breathing "no deeper than the second intercostal space" she managed to get home to her heating pad.

The pain subsided, and the next day Joan and another nurse went to San Francisco to a California Nurses' Association council meeting—a good place for a second, less severe attack. The third attack came on the Golden Gate bridge in rush-hour traffic.

Joan says, "I would have gone to any hospital, anywhere, if we could have gotten off that bridge." But the pain subsided before the traffic jam did, and she made it home. "Go to the Emergency Room at midnight for a pain I had for 35 hours? No way!" So Joan went to bed with her faithful heating pad, only to awaken at 5 A.M. "The knife again—the worst yet—so bad I couldn't sit up or reach the phone." She was drenched with perspiration and spitting up rusty, bloody sputum.

Joan's story ends with 16 days in the hospital, 6 weeks convalescence, and 6 months on anticoagulants.

Review 18

1. Most pulmonary emboli usually originate in the veins of the _____.

legs

2. Trace their route: They start in the legs, go to the _____ vena cava, right _____, right _____, and finally to a branch of the _____ artery.

inferior   atrium
ventricle   pulmonary

3. The clot doesn't pass through the lungs to the left atrium because _____ _____ _____ _____ _____.

pulmonary arteries are too small

4. If a small pulmonary artery branch is obstructed, there may be _____ _____ _____ symptoms.

no (or minor)

5. Obstruction of 50% or more of a main pulmonary artery leads to (hypertension/hypotension), circulatory _____, and death.

hypotension
collapse

Clinical Manifestations of Pulmonary Embolism (pp. 71–72)

Review 19

1. Pain from a pulmonary embolism usually (does/does not) radiate into the arms.

does not

2. The pain usually (is/is not) increased by deep inspiration.

is

3. In nearly all patients, the respiratory rate _____ and the heart rate _____.

increases
increases

4. With a stethoscope, you may hear _____ _____ _____.

wheezing or rales

5. You will need to order a _____ _____ and _____ _____ _____.

12-lead ECG   arterial blood gases

6. Radioactive _____ _____ is the best means of detecting a pulmonary embolism.

lung scanning

7. Because pulmonary emboli originate in the legs, you carefully evaluate every AMI patient for signs of _____.

thrombophlebitis

8. These signs include: _____, _____, and _____.

warmth   tenderness   swelling

9. The arterial blood gases will usually show _____.

hypoxemia

10. Twelve-lead ECG is of minimal help; it may show an acute strain pattern of the _____ heart.

right

11. The lung scan will show the segment of the lung that has been _____ ____ ____.

    deprived of O$_2$

12. Two times you will be especially aware of the dangers of pulmonary emboli are when Mr. Kardiak _____ _____ _____ and if he _____ _____ _____.

    first gets up   strains at stool

Cerebral Embolism *(pp. 72–73)*
Review 20

1. Clots originating in the left ventricle are called _____ thrombi.

   mural

2. Mural thrombi travel from the left _____ through the _____ to the _____ or _____ arteries.

   ventricle aorta cerebral peripheral

3. A cerebral embolus may cause the picture of a _____.

   stroke

4. Acute MI and a cerebral embolism = a _____ prognosis.

   poor

5. Why should an ECG be taken on patients admitted with a diagnosis of CVA?
   _____
   _____
   _____
   _____
   _____.

   Because the CVA may be due to an embolism after MI. With aphasia they couldn't describe the chest pain, etc., that preceded the stroke.

6. The symptoms of cerebral embolism occur (suddenly/gradually)

   suddenly

7. These may include _____ _____, _____, and _____ _____.

   motor weakness paralysis speech disturbance

8. A _____ scan may be used to diagnose a cerebral embolism.

   CAT

Peripheral Embolism *(p. 73)*
Review 21

1. Peripheral emboli most often lodge in the _____ or _____ arteries.

   femoral   iliac

2. Signs of a peripheral embolus are a _____, _____, _____ extremity.

   cold, pale, pulseless

3. If this occurs, you should promptly _____ _____ _____.

   notify the doctor

4. Immediate _____ may save the limb.

   surgery

5. Again, the best treatment of any kind of embolism is _____.

   prevention

Treatment of Thromboembolism *(pp. 73–74)*
Review 22

1. The best treatment of thromboembolism is _____ thrombi.

   preventing

2. Bedridden patients should receive low-dose subcutaneous _____ to prevent thrombosis.

   heparin

3. You would expect to see full-dose IV heparin after _____ therapy is started.

   thrombolytic

4. It would also be used if your patient exhibits (unstable/stable) angina.

   unstable

5. Mr. Kardiak's ECG shows a large anterior left ventricular infarction, you (would/would not) expect to use IV heparin.

   would

6. Venous stasis probably (increases/decreases) the chances of thrombus formation.

   increases

7. List two ways you can minimize venous stasis: _____ _____ _____, _____ _____ _____ _____ _____.

   turn patient periodically   regular passive leg and arm exercises

8. Elastic _____ are used to prevent _____ _____ check them for smooth fit.

   stockings   venous pooling

9. Elevating the gatch or placing pillows under the knees (is/is not) advisable. | is not

10. Drugs used to decrease clot formation are called _____. | anticoagulants

11. An overdose of anticoagulants may cause _____. | bleeding

12. Watch the patient closely for bleeding in _____, _____, or _____. | skin   urine   stools

13. Heparin is usually given in a constant _____ drip. | intravenous

14. Heparin is used to dissolve the embolus. (True/False) | False

15. Heparin is used to _____ _____ of the embolus. | prevent extension

16. A continuous heparin drip usually contains _____ units of heparin in 500 cc D_5W. | 20,000

17. The lab work ordered to check on clotting time will probably be an aPTT, that is, _____ _____ _____ time. | activated partial thromboplastin

18. Your patient's aPTT should be _____ to _____ the normal control value. | 2   2.5

19. You would expect the doctor to order an aPTT _____ to _____ hours after starting heparin and then _____. | 4   6 \ daily

20. If you are using a heparin lock rather than a drip, the usual dosage is _____ to _____ units every _____ to _____ hours. | 5000 \ 10,000   4   6

21. Heparin dosage is adjusted by the doctor in accordance with the patient's _____. | aPTT

22. The antidote (antagonist) for an overdose of heparin is _____ _____, or vitamin _____. | protamine sulfate \ K

Cardiac Tamponade *(pp. 74–75)*

Review 23

1. An AMI extending to the epicardial surface can cause inflammation of the _____. | pericardium

2. The pain of _____ (inflammation of the pericardium) is worsened by _____ _____ and changes in _____. | pericarditis \ deep breathing   position

3. Vital signs would show the patient has a _____. | fever

4. With your stethoscope you would hear a _____ sound with each heart beat; this is called a _____ _____ _____. | grating \ pericardial friction rub

5. You would expect to find a transient friction rub in about (1/4, 1/2, 3/4) of AMIs. | 1/2

6. Pericarditis usually (is/is not) serious. | is not

7. Extensively damaged myocardium may weaken and _____. | rupture

8. The rupture may take place in the _____ wall (or free wall) of the ventricle. | outer

9. Ventricular rupture is usually associated with extensive _____ infarction. | transmural

10. An outer wall rupture allows blood to leave the heart and fill the _____ ____. | pericardial sac

11. This rupture, which compresses or constricts the heart, is called _____ _____. | cardiac tamponade

12. This situation usually results in _____. | death

13. One third of the ventricular ruptures occur in the first _____ _____ with the first _____ showing the highest incidence of ruptures. | 2 days \ week

14. This occurs more often in (men/women) and in patients who were (hypertensive/hypotensive) before their AMI. | women   hypertensive

15. The patient may complain of _____, blood pressure _____, and the heart rate _____ abruptly. | pain   falls \ slows

16. The monitor may show _____ activity when the heart has stopped contracting.

    electrical

17. You should use _____ until the diagnosis of cardiac tamponade is determined.

    CPR

Take a really good look at Figure 5–6 (p. 70) in *The Manual*. It graphically depicts the complications of AMI. Can you visualize the progression you hope to prevent? Spend a few minutes studying it.

OTHER ASPECTS OF THE ACUTE PHASE OF MYOCARDIAL INFARCTION (p. 75)

Review 24

1. You expect temperature elevations. Temperature will rise about _____ _____ after AMI, remain elevated _____ to _____ days and usually be normal by the _____ day.

   24 hours
   2 3 5th

2. You expect a temperature of about _____°C.

   38

3. If Mr. Kardiak's fever is outside these limits, you watch for signs of _____, _____, or other infections.

   pneumonia
   thrombophlebitis

4. Chest pain usually is due to _____ _____ or _____ of the original MI.

   angina pectoris   extension

5. Be aware that _____ can also cause chest pain.

   pericarditis

6. Because recurrent pain indicates the acute process has _____ _____, you would perform _____ and _____ _____ after significant pain episodes.

   not stabilized
   ECG   enzyme studies

7. It is very important to give adequate pain _____, usually _____ _____.

   medication   morphine sulfate

Treatment During the Acute Phase (p. 75)
Review 25

1. Originally the treatment of AMI focused on reducing the myocardial _____ demand.

   oxygen

2. This is still important and to do this, you try to reduce physical and emotional _____ and give _____ _____.

   exertion   beta blockers

3. An aim of current treatment is to increase myocardial oxygen _____.

   supply

4. Drugs can be used to _____ _____ the clots and improve coronary perfusion.

   dissolve (lyse)

5. A procedure that unblocks obstructed arteries (you will learn more about it in Chapter 6) is called _____ _____ _____.

   percutaneous coronary
      angioplasty

THE RECOVERY PHASE OF MYOCARDIAL INFARCTION (pp. 75–76)

Review 26

1. Let's say that after two to three days Mr. Kardiak is in stable condition, the chances of complications now are (much decreased/the same/increased).

   much decreased

2. Initially, you restrict physical activity in order to _____ the heart's work; complete bedrest (is/is not) contraindicated.

   decrease
   is

3. List some of the advantages of early ambulation: _____ _____ _____ _____

   prevents cardiovascular decon-
   ditioning   prevents skeletal
   muscle wasting   helps avoid
   anxiety and depression

4. A cardiac rehabilitation program should include progressive _____, _____ about heart disease, and _____ on returning to a normal life.

   activity
   instruction   counseling

5. During the recovery phase, you must remember, _____ can occur at any time.

   complications

71

CRITICAL PATH FOR ACUTE MYOCARDIAL INFARCTION *(p. 76)*

Review 27

Study the Critical Path, Table 5–2 (pp. 78–79) in *The Manual*. This is for an "uncomplicated recovery." Now check your CCU. Are they using critical pathways? Keep in mind the goals of the critical path:

1. decrease _____ of care

2. improve _____ among health disciplines

3. provide _____ for quality assurance

4. _____ hospital stay

fragmentation

collaboration

data

decrease

HOSPITAL DISCHARGE *(pp. 76–77)*

Review 28

1. You can expect an AMI patient to remain in CCU about _____ days and be discharged from the hospital in _____ to _____ days.

2. Some clinical trials show that patients discharged _____ show no difference in morbidity or mortality.

3. To ensure safe, early mobilization, the doctor may order a _____ treadmill exercise test.

4. The _____ exercise increases the heart's rate _____ and helps to assess the patient's exercise _____.

5. Low-level exercise testing also helps predict the risk of _____ _____, recurrent _____, or _____ _____ for the next year or two.

6. Using a radioisotope, _____, with exercise testing increases the ability to predict high- and low-risk survivors.

7. This is called myocardial _____ imaging.

8. Predischarge exercise testing (is/is not) used on patients with complications.

3
7   10

earlier

low-level

low-intensity   moderately
tolerance

sudden death
AMI   angina pectoris

Thallium-201

perfusion

is not

DISCHARGE TEACHING *(p. 77)*

Review 29

Carefully compare Table 5–3 (p. 80) in *The Manual* to your hospital discharge teaching plan. You say there is no plan? Then get going, you have an ideal outline in Table 5.3.

1. It is vital that the patient understand and reduce _____ _____ for cardiac disease.

2. If the patient has a repeat AMI, research shows he (will/will not) get to the hospital sooner.

3. Mr. Kardiak and family must understand that getting to the hospital quickly allows _____ and saving of heart _____.

4. The procedure Mr. Kardiak should follow is to take _____ nitroglycerin _____ minutes apart and if no relief then call 911 or a special emergency number.

5. Mr. Kardiak should not take the time to call _____ _____.

6. Research shows that this _____ onset of treatment.

risk factors

will not

thrombolysis   muscle

3   3

his doctor

delays

7. Discharge activity instructions should cover a _____ program, return to sexual activity (usually within _____ to _____ weeks), and return-to-work schedule.

walking
2 3

8. Standard drug therapy includes low-dose _____ and _____ _____ therapy. (More on these later.)

aspirin   beta blocker

PROGNOSIS IN ACUTE MYOCARDIAL INFARCTION *(pp. 80–81)*

Review 30

1. Factors affecting the prognosis after an AMI are:

   a. _____ of infarct

   size

   b. _____

   location

   c. _____ of CAD

   extent

   d. _____ after onset

   complications

2. The most important determinant is very simply the _____ _____ of the heart after the AMI.

   pumping ability

3. If the left ventricular pumping ability is good, we say the patient has a normal _____ fraction.

   ejection

4. Ejection fraction is the _____ of blood emptied from the ventricle during contraction.

   percentage

5. Patients who have symptoms at rest and have a low ejection fraction (less than _____%) have an annual mortality rate of 50%.

   20

6. Of all AMIs discharged from the hospital, _____% will be dead at the end of one year.

   10

7. The best prognosis is for (younger/older) patients and patients with good _____ function.

   younger
   ventricular

6

Medical and Surgical Treatment
of Acute Myocardial Infarction

THE DEVELOPMENT OF INTENSIVE CORONARY CARE (pp. 83–85)

Review 1

1. In the "dark ages" of coronary care it was known that _____ _____ was responsible for 90% of arrhythmic deaths.

   ventricular fibrillation

2. Originally it was thought that ventricular fibrillation could only be treated with _____ electrical defibrillation (only possible during surgery).

   internal

Now let's organize the events leading up to where we are today. Put the events in chronological order.

DATES	EVENTS
1956 _____	A. Dr. Day at Bethany and Meltzer & Kitchell at Presbyterian-U of PA Medical Center start CCUs
1960 _____	B. Large-scale thrombolytic studies
1961 _____	C. Paul Zoll, external defibrillation
1962 _____	D. Meltzer & Kitchell study causes of death after AMI
1980 _____	E. Dr. Kouwenhaven, Johns Hopkins Hospital, develops CPR
mid-1980s _____	F. DeWood, thrombolytic therapy

Chronological Order

C, E, D, A, F, B

1. To get where we are today, required recognition that death results from the _____ of AMI.

   complications

2. Studies by Meltzer and Kitchell showed that about 50% of AMI deaths resulted from _____.

   arrhythmias

3. It was known that ventricular fibrillation, which caused 90% of all "sudden deaths," could be terminated by _____ _____.

   electric shock

4. The discovery (Paul Zoll, 1965) that defibrillation could be delivered _____ didn't help much because it had to be done within _____ to _____ minutes to be effective.

   externally
   1   2

5. Ventricular asystole (or standstill), the other sudden death arrhythmia, could be reversed by using a _____ within (seconds/minutes). (Neither were too useful when you had to wait 15 minutes or more for a doctor to come.)

pacemaker   seconds

6. In 1960 a procedure called _____ was developed to sustain circulation until medical treatment arrived but it required trained help immediately available.

CPR

7. In _____ CCUs were developed with specially educated _____ as the primary personnel.

1962   nurses

PHARMACOLOGIC TREATMENT OF ACUTE MYOCARDIAL INFARCTION (pp. 85–89)

Thrombolysis (pp. 85–86)
Review 2

1. Clots blocking the coronary arteries are present within _____ _____ of the onset of symptoms in _____% of all AMIs.

1 hour
90

2. Thrombolytic drugs work by _____ the clot and lowering the blood viscosity.

lysing (dissolving)

3. Thrombolytic drugs are involved with the activation of plasminogen to _____.

plasmin

4. Plasmin is an enzyme that breaks down _____, fibrinogen, and other procoagulant proteins into soluble fragments.

fibrin

5. Thrombolysis helps achieve three treatment goals:

a. _____

relieve pain and anxiety

b. _____

preserve myocardium

c. _____

prevent and treat complications

6. The most important factor in thrombolytic therapy is _____.

time

7. Considering that thrombi form within 1 hour of onset of symptoms, thrombolysis started within 1 hour of symptoms reduces mortality by _____%.

50

8. Thrombolysis within _____ hours of onset of symptoms reduces mortality by 23%.

3

9. Thrombolytic therapy (can/cannot) alter the course of AMI.

can

10. Thrombolysis started after _____ hours of onset of symptoms has no effect on mortality.

12

11. The least expensive thrombolytic is _____.

streptokinase

12. A sustained form of streptokinase is _____. (initials)

APSAC

13. The third thrombolytic is tissue plasminogen activator:

full name: _____

alteplase

initials: _____ or _____.

TPA   rt-PA

14. Learn all three thrombolytics, at least by their initials, you will meet many more drugs later.

15. Study Table 6–1 (p. 86, *The Manual*). Can you see where the dangers of thrombolysis could outweigh the benefits in both the "Relative and Absolute Contradindications"?

Alteplase (rt-PA)
Review 3

1. In studies, alteplase given over _____ minutes gave best results.

90

2. But alteplase after _____ hours was ineffective. (When the average delay time for getting treatment is 4 hours, you can see the problem.)

4

3. Let's make this as simple as possible: You need to start _____ IV lines, 2 of them _____-bore.

3
large

4. Simple: the standard rt-PA dose is _____ mg of rt-PA in _____ mL H$_2$O.   100   100

5. Therapy with rt-PA begins with a 15 mg IV _____ over 3 minutes.   bolus

6. You will need an _____ pump to administer 0.75 mg/kg over the next 30 minutes (up to _____ mg)   infusion   50

7. Slow the IV, and up to _____ mg of rt-PA is given over the next 60 minutes for a total of no more than _____ mg.   35   100

8. Fifty minutes after starting rt-PA, you give a bolus of 5000 U of _____.   heparin

9. You also start an IV _____ drip.   heparin

10. The heparin drip rate will be adjusted to achieve an _____ of 60 to 85 seconds.   APTT

11. PTT and activated clotting time will be measured every _____ _____.   6 hours

12. Heparin IV is continued for _____ hours and then tapered off.   48

13. rt-PA has a short half-life and can be _____ as needed.   readministered

Streptokinase
Review 4

1. Streptokinase is (more/less) expensive than rt-PA.   less

2. Trials have shown (a difference/no difference) in the outcomes between streptokinase and rt-PA.   no difference

3. Streptokinase is simply given IV drip _____ units in 100 ml D$_5$W over _____ hour.   1,500,000   1

Long-term Anticoagulation
Review 5

1. Long-term anticoagulation is accomplished with _____ or oral anticoagulants, eg, _____.   aspirin   warfarin

2. One study shows _____ as being better than _____; however, it causes more hemorrhagic complications.   warfarin   aspirin

Patient Assessment
Review 6

1. Vital signs are monitored _____.   q 15 minutes

2. Total _____ relief is vital.   pain

3. You do _____ checks to detect signs of intracranial hemorrhage.   neurologic

4. You test all stools for _____ _____.   occult blood

5. You watch the monitor carefully for _____ arrhythmias.   reperfusion

6. These result because the non-perfused areas of myocardium have built up _____ wastes, oxygen-free radicals, and _____.   metabolic   potassium

7. These are "washed out" with reperfusion and _____ may occur.   arrhythmias

8. Reinfarction can result from inadequate anticoagulation, so you watch the _____ results; baseline levels should be drawn every _____ hours.   APTT   12

9. If you adjust the heparin drip, you need a new APTT in _____ to _____ hours.   2   3

10. What are the four signs of reperfusion (ie, success!)?

   a. _____   relief of pain

   b. _____   reperfusion arrhythmias

c. _____

d. _____

reduction of ST segment eleva-
tion

peaking of CK-MB in less than
12 hours

11. Can you believe you will welcome an arrhythmia? However, you will treat very _____ or very _____ rate arrhythmias.

fast   slow

12. CK-MB will peak and begin dropping within _____ to _____ hours of reperfusion.

1   4

Review 7

If you have forgotten more than you ever knew about the autonomic nervous system and the drugs affecting it, you may be headed for deep water. Here is a life preserver, in the form of Review 7, to help you survive. (Pharmacology books will give you more information.)

Choose the right words from the pairs of words to fill in the blanks on the next page on the Autonomic Nervous System Chart.

AUTONOMIC NERVOUS SYSTEM
(Controls involuntary body functions)

Parasympathetic Nervous System
1A. (_____)

Sympathetic Nervous System
1B. (_____)

Sympathetic (Adrenergic) Receptors

(of special interest to ICCU)
2. alpha 1, alpha 2
3. beta 1 (heart)
4. beta 2 (bronchioles, arterioles)
5. dopamine1, dopamine 2

Effects of Stimulation on:

Parasympathetic Nervous System | Sympathetic Nervous System

6A. _____   6B. _____

7A. _____   7B. _____

8A. _____   8B. _____

9A. _____   9B. _____

10. Drug that increases an effect   _____

11. Drug that decreases an effect   _____

12. An antagonist is also called   _____

13. A suffix used to mean agonist   _____

14. A suffix used to mean blocker   _____

15. E.G., a sympathomimetic   _____

16. A sympatholytic   _____

17. A parasympathomimetic   _____

18. A parasympatholytic   _____

WORD PAIRS

1A, 1B:	adrenergic/cholinergic
6A, 6B:	vasoconstriction/vasodilation
7A, 7B, 8A, 8B:	decrease/increase
9A, 9B:	fight or flight/general slowing
10, 11:	agonist/antagonist
12:	augmenter/blocker
13, 14:	lytic/mimetic
15–18:	adrenergic/cholinergic; agonist/antagonist

ANSWERS

1A. cholinergic	1B. adrenergic
6A. vasodilation	6B. vasoconstriction
7A. decrease heart rate	7B. increase heart rate
8A. decrease blood pressure	8B. increase blood pressure
9A. general slowing	9B. fight or flight
10. agonist	11. antagonist
12. blocker	13. mimetic
14. lytic	15. adrenergic agonist
16. adrenergic antagonist	17. cholinergic agonist
18. cholinergic antagonist	

Nitrates *(p. 87)*
Review 8

1. Nitrates (nitroglycerin) increase _____ blood flow to ischemic myocardium.   — collateral

2. Nitrates (reduce/increase) the volume returning to heart (preload).   — reduce

3. They also (reduce/increase) the resistance the heart experiences (afterload).   — reduce

4. Nitrates are indicated in AMI complicated by _____ _____.   — heart failure

Beta Blockers *(p. 88)*
Review 9

1. Beta blockers are also called _____ drugs.   — anti-adrenergic

2. These drugs interfere with (or block) the effects of the _____ nervous system.   — sympathetic

3. Beta receptors are found in the _____ muscle, smooth muscle of the _____ system, and in the _____ tree.   — heart / vascular   bronchial

4. If beta receptors are stimulated (as opposed to blocked) the heart's ____ and _____ are increased. Also, systemic blood vessels and the bronchioles will _____.   — rate / contractility / dilate

5. Beta-1 receptors are found in the _____ and beta-2 receptors are found mainly in _____.   — heart / bronchioles

6. Beta-1 selective drugs tend to block _____ receptors and have less effect on _____ and _____ smooth muscles.   — heart / bronchial   vascular

7. Thus, the undesirable side effects of _____ and _____ will be less.   — bronchospasm / vasoconstriction

8. *The Manual* lists eight beta blockers, all of them end in the letters _____.   — OLOL

9. If you are in a CCU class and expected to memorize these, use this mnemonic for the beta-1 selective drugs:

*A b*eta *e*ffect on *m*yocardium

Write the drugs beginning with those letters below:

A = _____   B = _____   — atenolol   betaxolol

E = _____   M = _____   — esmolol   metoprolol

79

10. Non-selective beta blockers begin with the letters LNPT (I suppose that could stand for Licensed Nurse and Patient!)

L = _____   N = _____

P = _____   T = _____

labetolol   nadolol

propranolol   timolol

More on Betas
Review 10

1. Beta blockers are used with long-acting _____ to prevent _____ attacks and prevent myocardial _____.

nitrates   angina
ischemia

2. By blocking the sympathetic nervous system's effect, you decrease heart _____ and _____ and this (decreases/increases) the heart's work and its _____ demands.

rate
contractility   decreases
oxygen

3. Decreased heart rate prolongs (diastole/systole), which is when the _____ artery filling occurs and thus myocardial _____ is improved.

diastole   coronary
perfusion

4. Beta blockers also _____ the threshold at which _____ _____ will occur and this decreases the occurrence of sudden death.

increase (raise)   ventricular
fibrillation

Review 11

1. Beta blockers combined with thrombolytic drugs preserve _____ tissue during an AMI.

myocardial

2. Studies have shown a reduction in mortality when AMI patients are treated with beta blockers _____ to _____ hours after onset of symptoms.

4   5

3. Long-term beta blockade is suggested for all AMI patients who do not have severe heart _____ or _____ disease.

failure   lung

4. However, _____ AMIs with good _____ ventricular function do not appear to need or benefit from long-term beta-blocker therapy.

uncomplicated   left

Calcium-channel Blockers *(pp. 88–89)*
Review 12

1. Smooth muscle contraction depends on _____ ions.

calcium

2. If you block the entry of _____ ions through cell membranes you decrease contractions and _____.

calcium
spasms

3. Relaxing coronary arteries enables them to (dilate/constrict) and increase _____ blood flow and improve myocardial _____.

dilate   coronary
oxygenation

4. Thus calcium blockers (or calcium _____) can be effective in treating coronary artery _____, ie, _____ angina.

antagonists
spasm   variant

5. Calcium blockers are also effective in treatment of _____ angina.

stable

6. Calcium blockers have also been reported successful in treating resistant _____, heart _____ and hypertension.

arrhythmias
failure

7. Unfortunately, calcium blockers have not been found effective in treating _____.

AMI

8. Calcium blockers you may be familiar with are _____, _____, and _____.

verapamil   diltiazem
nifedipine

Angiotensin-converting-enzyme Inhibitors *(p. 89)*
Review 13

Take a quick look at Figure 7–4 (next chapter in *The Manual*). For right now, it's enough to know that this system works to increase both vasoconstriction and circulating blood volume. Not the best thing when we are trying to reduce the heart's work and decrease myocardial oxygen demand.

1. The classification of drugs used to block these adverse effects is called _____ _____ _____ _____.

   angiotensin-converting enzyme inhibitors

2. The three ACE inhibitors listed in *The Manual* all end in _____. (Remember the beta blockers ended in _____).

   OPRIL
   OLOL

3. Now, the three ACE inhibitors are _____, _____, and _____.

   captopril enalopril lisinopril

4. AMIs with ejection fractions less than ____% can benefit from these drugs.

   40

5. The evidence seems to be that these drugs improve survival and function in AMIs with _____ to _____ heart failure.

   moderate   severe

SUMMARY OF PHARMACOLOGIC TREATMENT FOR MYOCARDIAL INFARCTION *(p. 89)*

Review 14

1. There are three general areas of CCU treatment:

   a. prevent _____ _____ arrhythmias

   life threatening

   b. reduce myocardial _____ demand

   oxygen

   c. restore _____ flow to _____ myocardium

   blood   ischemic

   (C is also known as "salvage ischemic areas.")

2. For best results, pharmacotherapy must begin within _____ hour of symptom onset.

   1

3. Within 15 to 30 minutes of hospitalization begin _____ therapy.

   thrombolytic

4. Fifty minutes after that therapy is started, begin _____ therapy with full-dose IV _____.

   anticoagulant
   heparin

5. _____ _____ are used to reduce myocardial oxygen consumption and salvage _____ myocardium.

   Beta blockers
   ischemic

6. _____ _____ inhibitors are used to treat patients with left ventricular failure.

   angiotensin-converting enzyme

CORONARY REVASCULARIZATION *(pp. 89–93)*

Review 15

1. The majority of AMIs who could benefit from thrombolytic therapy don't receive it. Why? _____
   _____
   _____

   delay too long before coming to hospital

2. Two other techniques used for coronary _____ (increasing blood supply) are (initials, please) _____ and _____.

   revascularization
   PTCA   CABG

3. Just once write out each of those and then we will be happy to use the initials: _____
   _____

   See The Manual, p. 90

4. These procedures are not used routinely on all AMI patients prior to discharge but are used for patients who have _____.

   restenosis

Review 16

Read the information on page 90 in *The Manual* and study Figure 6–1. Close *The Manual* and draw your own picture of an obstructed artery.

1. Got your large catheter, called a _____ catheter, ready?

   guiding

2. You will insert it into either a _____ or _____ artery and pass it to the _____ of the involved vessel.

   femoral   brachial
   ostium

3. With coronary _____, you visualize the exact location of the stenotic area.

4. Now insert the smaller catheter, the coronary _____ catheter, to the site of the _____.

5. Pass the short, flexible guidewire in through the obstruction and _____ the balloon for _____ to _____ seconds.

6. Have you drawn it? You have just squished (okay, _____) the plaque and unblocked the artery.

angiography
dilatation
obstruction (plaque)
inflate
3   5
compressed

Advantages and Disadvantages
Review 17

1. With PTCA there should be an immediate increase in coronary _____ _____ without the dangers of _____ and anesthesia.

2. The dangers of PTCA are the possibility of occlusion due to dissection, _____, or _____.

3. Thus a cardiac surgical team needs to be available for emergency _____ surgery.

4. PTCA is most useful in patients with (one/more than one) blocked vessel.

5. After successful PTCA, the in-hospital reocclusion rate is (significantly better/worse) than with thrombolytic therapy.

6. The bad news, _____ to _____% of PTCA patients will eventually need another procedure because of restenosis and recurring _____.

blood flow
surgery
thrombus
spasm
bypass
one
significantly better
25   50
angina

New Developments in the Treatment
of Coronary Stenosis *(pp. 91–93)*
Review 18

There are five new procedures described that replace PTCA or serve as an adjunct to it. They are listed here with a Roman numeral for you to use in the exercise. You can sort out some of the information about each technique by matching it to the correct statement.

Revascularization techniques:
I = directional atherectomy, II = transluminal extraction endarterectomy, III = rotational atherectomy (Rotablator), IV = laser ablation, V = angioplasty stents

Matching exercise

Devices:

continuous vacuum suction of debris _____

pulses of ultraviolet or infrared light _____

implantable metallic tube _____

rigid housing, rotating blade, collection chamber _____

diamond coated abrasive tip _____

II
IV
V
I
III

Indication/Contraindications:

contraindication = heavily calcified, stiff vessels _____

indication = long, diffuse lesions, small tortuous vessels _____

indication = old saphenous vein grafts _____

indication = long, diffuse lesions, old vein grafts _____

I
III
II
IV

Restenosis rates:

25% restenosis rate (with PTCA) _____   V

restenosis similar to PTCA (25 to 50%) _____   I

39% restenosis rate _____   III

46% restenosis rate _____   II

Miscellaneous:

complications: vascular injury, bleeding 16% _____   V

rotates at 2500 rpm _____   II

rotates at 200,000 rpm _____   III

should leave smooth surface, less clots _____   I

high success rate with difficult lesions _____   IV

Nursing Care (*p. 93*)
Review 19

1. You would prepare a revascularization patient the same as you do a patient for _____ _____.   cardiac catheterization

2. Patient and family need _____ and reassurance about the procedure and aftermath.   teaching

3. After the procedure, it is important to assess _____ signs, especially _____ pulses for signs of _____ or hematoma at the _____ _____ site.   vital   distal   thrombosis   arterial puncture

4. You also carefully monitor _____ and _____ status.   cardiac   hemodynamic

5. The contrast dye used will be excreted through the _____ so you would (encourage/discourage) fluid intake.   kidneys   encourage

SURGICAL TREATMENT (*p. 93*)
Review 20

Ready to try a few questions about coronary artery bypass graft? (To save space, we will call it CABG.)

1. In CABG a portion of the patient's _____ vein or internal mammary artery is used for the graft.   saphenous

2. The atherosclerotic process usually involves (one/two or more) coronary arteries and that determines the number of grafts.   two or more

3. CABG is most effective when: (a) atherosclerosis is diffuse, (b) narrowing of the artery is near the point of origin. (Choose one.)   b

Review 21

Label the following statements YES if they are correct statements in reference to CABG. Label them NO if they are false.

a. costs less than PTCA _____   a. no

b. relieves stable angina _____   b. yes

c. increases exercise tolerance _____   c. yes

d. stops progression of CAD _____   d. no

e. reduces heart failure _____   e. yes

f. effective in right coronary and LAD artery disease _____ | f. yes

g. better functional than PTCA _____ | g. yes

h. relieves unstable angina _____ | h. yes

i. fewer complications than PTCA _____ | i. yes

j. less risk than PTCA _____ | j. no

Review 22

Your patient, Mr. Angie Peck, has been admitted for surgery to receive a coronary artery bypass graft. Dr. Brusque, world-renowned coronary surgeon, spent 32 seconds yesterday explaining the procedure to the Pecks. He can't understand why they still have questions, but, because he is in surgery all day, he asks you to talk with them. He tells you, "I explained everything yesterday, but go ahead and answer any questions they have." Try to imagine yourself in the scene below and complete the nurse's explanation.

As you enter the visitor's waiting room, you are pounced upon.

Mrs. Pyranna: I'm the daughter. When's that Dr. Brusque going to talk to us? We've been waiting here for hours.

Nurse: You've done a lot of waiting these last few days, haven't you? You must be worn out. Let's all sit down and I'll see if I can help.

Mrs. Pyranna: Dr. Brusque, is he . . ?

Nurse: Dr. Brusque is sorry he couldn't see you this morning. He's in surgery. He has another patient who needed the same type of surgery that Mr. Peck is scheduled for. Dr. Brusque asked me to answer questions you may have about the coronary artery bypass grafts. Do you have anything you would like to ask me about?

Mrs. Peck: (sniffling) It seems so frightening—dangerous—cutting into the heart and . . . and all for *what?* It's not going to cure him, is it?

Nurse: There still is _____ _____ for coronary heart disease. Of the people who have this surgery _____% feel much better afterward. By this I mean,

_____

_____

_____

| no cure
| 85
| they can live a more normal life without having the heart pain they had before surgery.

Mrs. Pyranna: Percents don't mean anything to Ma.

Nurse: Mrs. Peck, let me explain the 85% this way. _____

_____

_____

| If 10 people had this type of surgery, 8, perhaps 9, of those people would feel much better after surgery.

Mrs. Pyranna: If Dad has this surgery, will it increase his chances for living longer?

Nurse: I wish I could give you a definite answer on that. _____

_____

| We need more research and experience before we have definite answers.

Mrs. Pyranna: How do they do this surgery? Dr. Brusque said they take a vein from the leg and sew it into the heart. That's not going to work. They'd have to pull an awful lot of vein up to reach clear to his heart.

Nurse: Maybe I can draw a picture that would help. But first let me explain about the leg vein. _____

_____

_____

_____

_____

_____

| The surgeon cuts a small piece of vein out of the leg and sews it into the artery in the heart that is blocked. It's like a detour—the blood can flow through the new piece of vein and avoid the blockage.

Mrs. Peck: Oh dear, he'll be in a wheelchair the rest of his life. The would just kill him.

Nurse: Oh, no, Mrs. Peck. There are plenty of other veins to supply his leg. Look at your own leg and you will see lots of veins.

7

Heart Failure

Review 1

1. Heart failure means that the injured _____ is unable to pump enough blood to meet the _____ needs of the body.

   myocardium
   metabolic

2. *The Manual* (p. 95), lists nine conditions associated with heart failure. See how many you can list and check them with page 95, paragraph 1.

3. With an aging population, you will see more heart failure patients; in fact, _____ out of _____ people over 75 years has heart failure.

   1
   10

VENTRICULAR FUNCTION AND CARDIAC OUTPUT *(pp. 95–96)*

Review 2

1. Ventricles fill. Ventricles pump out the blood. Do they pump out 100% of the blood they received (healthy ventricles that is)? _____

   no

2. How much of their total volume is normally pumped out? _____

   60 to 70%

3. This figure is called the _____ _____.

   ejection fraction

4. A patient with heart failure will have an ejection fraction of less than _____%.

   40

5. In Chapter 5 you learned that patients with _____ _____ below 20% had a mortality rate exceeding 50%.

   ejection fractions

Review 3

Now let's take a good look at stroke volume, preload, afterload, and contractility.

1. When the ventricle fills and dilates, its muscle fibers stretch or _____.

   lengthen

2. The more the fibers _____, the harder they can contract. (If you doubt this, stretch a rubber band a bit and snap yourself, then stretch it a lot and snap yourself. Convinced?)

   lengthen

3. The degree to which muscle fibers can shorten is called _____.

   contractility

4. Contractility is (based on/independent of) preload and afterload.

   independent of

5. Preload is the _____ of ventricular myocardial _____ present at the on-set of systole (contraction).

degree   stretch

6. Or to restate that, it is the end-_____ _____ or pressure.

diastolic volume

7. You can measure that! How? _____

PCWP

8. Now, afterload is the force against which the _____ contracts in _____.

myocardium
systole

9. Afterload is measured by _____ vascular resistance.

systemic

10. The combined effects of contractility, preload, and afterload determine the _____ of blood pumped from the ventricle with each contraction.

volume

11. And the volume pumped with each contraction is called _____ _____.

stroke volume

12. Stroke volume refers to the volume of each _____. And cardiac output is the _____ volume of blood pumped per _____.

contraction
total   minute

13. So the logical equation is:

cardiac output = _____ _____ × _____ _____.

stroke volume   heart rate

Review 4

Do a Matching exercise just to be sure you have these terms straight. There are six terms labeled A through F. And there are fifteen statements. Place the correct statement numbers under each term.

A. Ejection fraction

_____

D. Afterload

_____

B. Contractility

_____

E. Stroke volume

_____

C. Preload

_____

F. Cardiac output

_____

STATEMENTS

1. not based on preload and afterload

2. force against which myocardium contracts

3. 60 to 70% of total is normal

4. stroke volume × heart rate

5. amount of blood pumped compared to amount received

6. degree of myocardial stretch at onset of systole

7. degree to which muscle fibers can shorten

8. volume pumped with each systole

9. end-diastolic volume or pressure

10. less than 40% = heart failure

11. measured by systemic vascular resistance

12. half of cardiac output equation

13. measured by PCWP

14. total volume pumped per minute

15. combined effects of contractility, preload, and afterload

ANSWERS

A = 3, 5, 10

B = 1, 7

C = 6, 9, 13

D = 2, 11

E = 8, 12, 15

F = 4, 14

COMPENSATORY MECHANISMS (pp. 96–98)

Review 5

1. A sympathetic nervous system reflex is triggered by (decreased/increased) cardiac output.

decreased

2. The sympathetic nervous system causes the heart rate to _____ and strength of myocardial _____ to increase.

increase
contraction

3. _____ _____ diastolic pressure increases due to residual volume.

Ventricular end

4. This _____ the muscles and, at least initially, _____ cardiac output (Frank–Starling mechanism).

stretches   increases

Renin–Angiotensin–Aldosterone System (p. 97)
Review 6

1. _____ cardiac output also triggers the renin–angiotensin–aldosterone system.

Low

2. The juxtaglomerular cells of the _____ are affected by _____ renal perfusion to secrete _____.

kidneys   decreased
renin

3. Renin acts on circulating _____ to form angiotensin I which then forms _____ II.

angiotensinogen
angiotensin

4. Angiotensin II is a _____ and it helps to maintain _____ _____.

vasoconstrictor
blood pressure

5. Angiotensin II also stimulates the _____ mechanism and this would encourage increased fluid intake.

thirst

6. The decreased renal perfusion stimulates the _____ to produce the hormone _____.

adrenals
aldosterone

7. Aldosterone acts to retain _____ and _____ and thus (decrease/increase) circulating blood volume.

sodium   water   increase

Antidiuretic Hormone (pp. 97–98)
Review 7

1. Antidiuretic hormone is secreted to increase water _____ and _____ circulating blood volume.

retention   increase

2. An increase in blood volume is intended to _____ ventricular end-diastolic pressure and thus increase _____ volume.

increase
stroke

3. The three compensatory mechanisms (see Fig. 7–4, p. 98 in *The Manual*) are the body's attempt to counteract the effects of _____ _____.

heart failure

4. But after a certain point they become deleterious and overt heart failure develops, this stage is called _____.

decompensation

PATHOPHYSIOLOGY OF LEFT HEART FAILURE (pp. 98–99)

Review 8

1. The failing left ventricle pumps less blood with each contraction and empties (completely/incompletely).

incompletely

2. The left ventricle pumps blood into the _____ circulation.

systemic

3. Blood returns to the left ventricle from the lungs through the _____ _____ into the left atrium.

pulmonary
veins

4. When returning blood enters the partly full and failing left ventricle, the pressure _____ during diastole.

rises

5. This is known as increased _____ _____ _____.

ventricular diastolic pressure

6. This increase in left ventricular pressure causes a back pressure in the _____ _____ and in the _____ _____.

left atrium
pulmonary veins

7. The increased pulmonary venous pressure forces _____ from the capillaries into the lung tissues.

fluid

8. The very first stage of impending left ventricular failure is (increased/decreased) pressure in the pulmonary veins.

increased

9. Initially the increased pulmonary venous pressure (does/does not) produce symptoms.

does not

10. Further pulmonary venous hypertension may force _____ from the capillaries into the tissues surrounding the alveoli of the lungs.

fluid

11. This fluid is called _____ edema.

interstitial

12. Interstitial edema means there is fluid in the tissues _____ _____ _____.

around the alveoli

13. Interstitial edema (does/does not) cause symptoms.

does not

14. But it can be diagnosed on _____ _____.

chest x-ray

15. Alveolar edema causes definite symptoms and is diagnosed as _____ left ventricular failure.

overt

CLINICAL MANIFESTATIONS OF LEFT VENTRICULAR FAILURE (pp. 99–102)

Review 9

1. With alveolar edema the patient has the symptom of _____.

dyspnea

2. Since mild dyspnea is difficult to observe, you should ask if the patient _____ _____ _____ _____.

feels short
 of breath

3. Requests by the patient to elevate the head of the bed may indicate the form of dyspnea called _____.

orthopnea

4. When the patient suffers from dyspnea while lying flat, this shortness of breath is termed _____.

orthopnea

Paroxysmal Nocturnal Dyspnea (p. 100)

I wish that while you are studying this, you could actually take care of patients with left ventricular failure. Then the words on page 100 of *The Manual* would come alive for you. If you have any patients with this diagnosis, try to spend some time observing them. As a poor secondbest, I will tell you about two patients I remember. Would you please join me on the night shift of the day this actually happened?

We were only halfway through our CCU course, incompetent, unready, but inescapably there. Cardiac patients seemed to be everywhere, but our CCU wasn't ready yet. In desperation we gathered the patients and emergency supplies into a six-bed ward, a cardiac ward.

"Mr. Kardiak had a quiet evening. No complaints. Asleep by 10." The P.M. nurse closed the Kardex and went home. The shadows settled down on our makeshift set-up.

Twelve o'clock and all was . . . Was that a small cough? Suddenly Mr. Kardiak launches himself bolt upright in bed, wheezing, choking, clutching his chest, shaking the side rails. He coughs and sneezes and gasps, "Can't breathe—air—window."

I run to his bed, stumbling over the oxygen tank. The pain in my ankle activates my brain. "This oxygen will do you more good than the window. You'll be able to breathe easier with it on," I say as you quickly turn on the tank and together we strap on his mask. "If you sit still, you'll need less air," I tell him. "We'll put the side rails down and help you sit on the edge of the bed if you promise not to run for the window."

You drop the side rail and we support him on the edge of the bed. Even though he is panting and purple, we reassure him, and in a few minutes (that seems like hours) his dyspnea eases.

Finally, he collapses into sleep and we collapse at our desk. We have just handled our first case of paroxysmal nocturnal dyspnea (PND).

Review 10

1. Explain the term *paroxysmal nocturnal dyspnea.*

   Paroxysmal because _____.   the attack starts suddenly

   Nocturnal because _____.   it usually occurs at night

   Dyspnea because _____.   the main symptom is marked shortness of breath

2. Although PND occurs suddenly, the patient has probably had _____ _____ left ventricular failure first.   incipient (or subclinical)

3. If the patient wants to sit up, you should _____.   let him sit up

4. The most effective way of giving this patient oxygen is _____.   with a face mask

5. Obviously, the patient is frightened by this terrifying experience. What can you do about this? _____ _____.   Talk to him and reassure him that the attack will soon pass

6. PND results from decompensation of the _____ _____ after an acute increase in pulmonary _____ congestion.   left ventricle
venous

Physical Signs *(p. 100)*
Review 11

1. If Mr. Kardiak is suffering from moderate heart failure there may be (some/no) physical findings.   no

2. As the severity of the disease progresses, you auscultate carefully for _____, which are present in about one third of patients with heart failure.   rales

3. You may find a _____ heart sound in about two thirds of the patients with heart failure.   3rd

Rales *(p. 100)*
Review 12

1. Rales are abnormal breath sounds caused by fluid in the _____.   alveoli

2. As the disease progresses, the rales progress from _____ to _____ in the lung fields.   basilar   higher

3. With acute pulmonary edema, you will find rales, described as _____ and _____; they will be (high in the chest/throughout the lung fields).   coarse   bubbling
throughout the lung fields

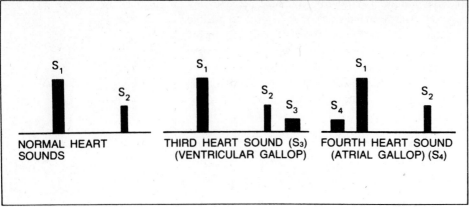

Figure 7.1. Normal heart sounds and components of a gallop rhythm. (from Meltzer et al. 4th ed.)

Third and Fourth Heart Sounds/Apical Impulse *(p. 100)*
Review 13

You have never heard a ventricular gallop? How do you identify one? First, listen closely to many normal hearts; get used to the S_1 and S_2 sounds. After you have become familiar with normal heart sounds, read the doctor's notes and listen in during report to discover those patients who have a ventricular gallop. Take your stethoscope to the patient and

1. Listen carefully to the two normal heart sounds; they are called _____ and _____. S_1 S_2

2. To hear a gallop rhythm, place the (bell/diaphragm) of your stethoscope over the _____ of the heart. bell / apex

3. If it is a ventricular gallop rhythm, you will hear an extra sound (before/after) the (first/second) sound. after / second

4. This is called an _____ sound. S_3

5. Sometimes you may also hear an extra sound that comes just before S_1. This is an _____ gallop. atrial

6. Rather than call this a pre-S_1, it is termed an _____ gallop. S_4

7. S_4 is (more/less) serious than S_3. less

8. An S_3 indicates _____ of the left ventricle. dilation

9. Thus, an S_3 is a definite sign of _____ _____ _____. left ventricular failure

10. Find the 5th intercostal space and draw a line down from the midline of the clavicle. Where they intersect you should find the _____ _____. apical impulse

11. When the heart enlarges, as in heart failure, the impulse shifts toward the (right/left). left

Treatment of Left Ventricular Failure *(pp. 101–102)*
Review 14

1. The best approach to treating left ventricular failure is _____ _____ and prompt treatment, especially with the drugs classified as _____ _____. early detection / ACE inhibitors

2. One aim of the drug therapy is to reduce the _____ of the heart and improve _____ efficiency. workload / pumping

3. _____ devices (eg, intraaortic balloon pumping or external counterpulsation) may be used, especially in cardiogenic shock, to improve left ventricular _____. Mechanical / function

90

4. Emergency _____ surgery (CABG) is a surgical treatment option.

bypass

5. To summarize questions 1 through 4: Four treatment approaches for left ventricular failure are _____ _____, _____ _____, _____ _____, and _____.

early detection   drug therapy
mechanical devices   surgery

6. The objective of all treatments is to _____ _____ _____.

increase cardiac output

Review 15

1. The overall objective in treating left ventricular failure is _____ _____ _____.

increasing
   cardiac output

2. To do that, we work with the four principal mechanisms in Figure 7.2. Fill in the top blanks labeled I through IV.

3. When the doctor orders drugs or treatments for our patient with acute heart failure, it helps to relate them to the four mechanisms of Figure 7.2. So let's complete the rest of the blanks in that diagram with the next five exercises.

I. Preload _____   II. Afterload _____   III. Myocardial _____
Rx obj. _____   Rx obj. _____   Rx obj. _____
Rx used: Rx used: Rx used:
   1. _____   1. _____   1. _____
   2. _____

I. Volume   II. Resistance
III. Contractility   IV. Rate

IV. Stroke Volume _____   V. Heart _____
Rx obj. _____   Rx obj. _____
Rx used: _____   ×   Rx used: _____   =
      1. _____

CARDIAC OUTPUT

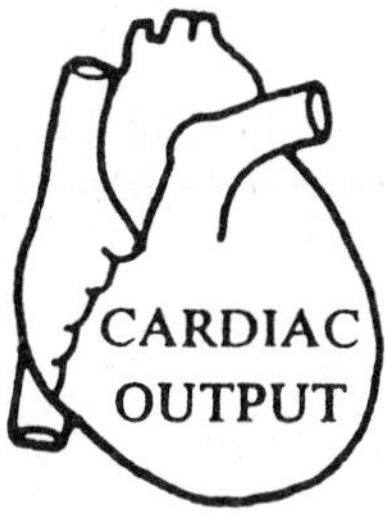

Figure 7.2

Mechanism I—Preload Volume

1. The objective is to (decrease/increase) preload volume, or as the therapy is called, preload volume _____.

decrease
reduction

(Write the three words of your last answer in the blank labeled *Rx. obj.* under I in Figure 7.2.)

2. Here we go with the increase/decrease mechanisms again. Put your choice (increases/decreases) in the blanks. Preload volume reduction _____ filling of the left ventricle, _____ pulmonary venous pressure, and thus _____ stroke volume, _____ cardiac output, and _____ pulmonary venous congestion.

decreases
decreases
increases   increases   decreases

3. Drugs used to increase urinary output and decrease blood volume are _____. (Write your answer in under *I, Rx. used;* 1 (Fig. 7.2).

diuretics

91

4. Drugs used to dilate or relax peripheral blood vessels are called _____. (Write your answer in under *I, Rx. used;* 2 (Fig. 7.2).

> vasodilators

5. Vasodilators can dilate the _____ system, the _____ system, or both.

> venous arterial

6. _____ inhibitors are vasodilators that reduce both _____ and _____. (Write your answers in under *Rx. obj.* in the correct spaces.)

> ACE preload
> afterload

7. Examples of ACE inhibitors are _____ and _____.

> enalopril captopril

8. They block the conversion of angiotensin I to _____. (See Fig. 7–4 in *The Manual.*)

> angiotensin II

9. They also _____ aldosterone levels and thus decrease _____ volume. (Again Fig. 7–4 says it better than words.)

> decrease intravascular

10. ACE inhibitors have been shown to (1) _____ heart failure after AMI, (2) reduce _____ in patients with heart failure, and (3) improve _____ status in patients with advanced heart failure.

> prevent
> mortality
> functional

11. ACE inhibitors should be used in patients with ejection fractions under _____%.

> 40

12. ACE inhibitors should be standard therapy in all patients with _____ _____.

> heart
> failure

13. The desired results of the vasodilator, nitroglycerin, would be venous _____ of the blood.

> pooling

14. To summarize: in treating left ventricular failure you may give your patients drugs that are classified as _____ or _____ to achieve _____ _____ _____.

> diuretics vasodilators
> preload volume reduction

15. ACE inhibitors are _____ that affect both _____ volume and _____ resistance.

> vasodilators preload
> afterload

Mechanism II—Afterload Resistance

1. The second method of treatment for advanced heart failure is afterload _____. (Write the two words in your answer in the blank labeled *Rx. obj.* under II in Figure 7.2.)

> reduction

2. Treatment of afterload resistance is designed to decrease the _____ or _____ against which the heart must pump.

> pressure
> resistance

3. High arterial pressure (decreases/increases) stroke volume and (decreases/increases) the heart's work.

> decreases increases

4. _____ vasodilators may be used to decrease afterload resistance.

> Arterial

5. ACE inhibitors may be chosen because they decrease both _____ volume and _____ resistance.

> preload
> afterload

6. Add two more drugs to your drug vocabulary: listed in *The Manual* are _____ and _____.

> prazosin
> nitroprusside

7. Prazosin is an alpha antagonist, or a sympath_____, which causes vaso-_____ and _____ mean arterial blood pressure.

> olytic
> dilation decreases

8. Nitroprusside is a nonnitrate vaso_____ with effects similar to nitrates.

> dilator

Mechanism III—Myocardial Contractility

1. The objective of treatment of this mechanism is to _____ _____ _____. (Write the three words of your answer in the blank labeled *Rx. obj.* under III in Fig. 7.2.)

> increase myocardial
>   contractility

2. If you can strengthen myocardial contractility, you will (increase/decrease) ventricular emptying, and thus the blood left in the ventricle (residual volume) should (increase/decrease).

> increase
>
> decrease

3. This should improve stroke _____ and cardiac _____.   volume   output

4. _____ drugs (eg, digitalis or amrinone) are a traditional heart failure treatment that is now being questioned. (Write your answer in on Fig. 7.2.)   Inotropic

5. With inotropic therapy, increased myocardial _____ _____ is the price of the increased contractility and may lead to (increased/decreased) morbidity and mortality.   oxygen consumption increased

6. Inotropics (should/should not) be used in the earliest stages of AMI.   should not

7. Dangerous complications to watch for with digitalis therapy are _____ and increased energy expenditure of the heart.   arrhythmias

Mechanism IV—Stroke Volume

1. Stroke volume is dependent on numbers _____, _____, and _____.   I II III

2. The treatment objective is to _____ the volume pumped with each stroke. (Write this in on Fig. 7.2.)   increase

3. The treatment used would be anything that positively affects numbers _____, _____, and _____. (See how easy this is?)   I II III

Mechanism V—Heart Rate

1. Heart rates that are too _____ or too _____ result in decreased cardiac _____.   fast slow output

2. The objective of the treatment of this mechanism is to _____ the heart _____. (Write the four words of your answer in the blank labeled *Rx. obj.* under V in Fig. 7.2.)   regulate rate

3. Fast rates don't allow time for the ventricles to _____ and thus decrease _____.   fill volume

4. Slow rates decrease cardiac _____ because of their infrequency.   output

5. Drugs or cardiac _____ may be used to regulate the heart's rate. (Write the two words of your answer in blank V.1. in Fig. 7.2.)   pacing

6. And now for the final equation:

Stroke volume × heart rate = _____ _____   cardiac output

ACUTE PULMONARY EDEMA (pp. 103–104)

Now if you have had a short break, won't you come back to our Cardiac Unit? Did I mention we had one empty bed? Well, Dr. Hart is going to remedy that; he has just called from ER with a direct admit. I'm scared. Dr. Hart sounded frantic!

The phone is still warm when he crashes through the door with the stretcher, and with one quick move we transfer his emergency patient to Bed 1. He says, "We'll need oxygen, an IV, morphine, a Foley, a diuretic, aminophylline, and maybe digitalis." Then he whispers, "He's moribund."

I fix the drugs while you help the patient. Our emergency is a miniature Santa Claus: white hair, white mustache, and an adorable goatee. (He really *did* exist.) But his beard is ·covered with a creeping, crawling, bubbling foam, a frothy mucus that pours incessantly out of his nose and mouth and nearly engulfs him. He is coughing, drowning, and is too weak to protest, so you continually wipe the mucus, give him oxygen, and try to calm him as you attach the monitor. Meanwhile, Dr. Hart is pawing through our emergency drugs. I plop his favorite IV intercath in his hands and tell him, "If you'll start the IV, here's your morphine and here's the aminophylline . . ." I'm halfway through when he decides to use digitalis. I flop a Foley cath set onto the bed and make another grab into the medicine cart. Dr. Hart inserts the IV, and I slowly give the drugs.

You leave the mucus tide to check the BP. You look up, shake your head, and try again. Dr. Hart swears at the monitor. Aren't you glad you can't interpret arrhythmias yet? Through all the confusion, I hear the purr of your voice as you reassure Santa Claus.

Gradually, the pace slows and we all begin to smile. Santa Claus is asleep when we open his chart. Dr. Hart writes his orders, then says: "When I came through that door, I had no idea we could save him." He smiles a goodnight. We have just successfully treated acute pulmonary edema.

Review 16

Now let's relate the treatment of acute pulmonary edema to our Santa Claus.

Point 1

1. "Santa Claus," or any acute pulmonary edema patient, should be placed in _____ position. — Fowler's

2. This encourages blood to pool in the _____ _____ and (decreases/increases) venous return. — lower body   decreases

Point 2

1. Morphine is used to reduce anxiety and to _____ the brain's respiratory center. — depress

2. This helps (decrease/increase) the respiratory rate. — decrease

3. Morphine also decreases preload volume by its _____ effect on peripheral veins. — vasodilator

Point 3

1. Alveolar edema (increases/decreases) the available space for air in the lungs. — decreases

2. Therapy with _____ helps to increase the concentration of oxygen available to the alveoli. — oxygen

3. The nasal cannula is the (most/least) effective means of administering oxygen. — least

4. If necessary, oxygen can be given using an _____ machine. — IPPB

Point 4

1. _____ are drugs that help the body eliminate excess fluids. — Diuretics

2. Two rapid-acting IV diuretics are _____ and _____. — Lasix   Edecrin

3. Their generic names are _____ and _____ _____. — furosemide   ethacrynic acid

4. Theoretically, they (increase/decrease) elimination of extracellular fluid. — increase

5. This, in turn, (increases/decreases) the blood volume returning to the heart, which then (increases/decreases) pulmonary venous pressure and reduces edema. — decreases decreases

6. These drugs also seem to cause the _____ to dilate and hold more blood thus (reducing/increasing) pulmonary edema even before the diuresis occurs. — veins reducing

Point 5

1. Vasodilators promote "pooling" of the blood and thus _____ preload volume. — reduce

2. The venous dilator _____ 0.4 to 0.8 mg sublingually can relieve dyspnea in 2 to 3 minutes. — nitroglycerin

3. The generic name for longer-lasting, slow-onset nitrates used to decrease pulmonary edema is _____ _____. — isosorbide dinitrate

4. Two isosorbide dinitrates you might find in your CCU are _____ and _____. (Do not confuse with isosorbide, an oral osmotic diuretic.) — Isordil Sorbitrate

5. Two vasodilators that work on both venous and arterial networks are _____ and _____. — nitroprusside prazosin

6. Of the four mechanisms, _____ _____ is the most difficult to treat.

heart rate

7. During vasodilator therapy, we watch patients for the complications of _____ and postural _____.

headaches hypotension

Point 6

1. Bronchodilators are used to relieve _____.

bronchospasm

2. The most common bronchodilator is _____, dosage _____ to _____ mg given IV.

aminophylline 250 500

3. Aminophylline's beneficial actions include _____ bronchioles, _____ cardiac output, and _____ venous pressure.

dilating increasing decreasing

4. Aminophylline's side effects may be _____ and _____.

hypotension arrhythmias

5. Suppose Dr. Halforder calls and says: "Give aminophylline 250 mg IV stat and repeat prn." How would you give it? Check all correct notations below:

A. undiluted
B. dilute to 50 cc
C. dilute to 100 cc
D. in 500 cc D₅W
E. fast push
F. over 5 minutes
G. over 10 minutes
H. over 15 minutes

B and H

The prn repeat is usually:

A. every 30 to 60 minutes
B. every 1 to 2 hours
C. every 3 to 4 hours
D. every 6 to 8 hours

C

RIGHT HEART FAILURE (pp. 104–107)

So far we have been talking about the left side of the heart. Now we take a look at the right side. Before starting, go back and review Figure 7–1 in *The Manual*. Try to imagine a force or pressure pushing the blood backwards through the left heart, the lungs, and the right heart. Oversimplified, yes, but understandable.

Review 17

1. After an MI, (left/right) heart failure is most common.

left

2. Left heart failure causes pulmonary venous pressure to _____.

rise

3. So when the right heart tries to empty, it meets increased pressure in the pulmonary _____.

circulation

4. Therefore, pulmonary artery pressure also _____.

rises

5. The right ventricle then (does/does not) empty completely.

does not

6. Then blood entering the right atrium meets (increased/decreased) pressure.

increased

7. This causes _____ back pressure within the entire peripheral venous system.

increased

8. Low renal perfusion results from _____ left ventricular output, ie, (forward/backward) heart failure.

decreased forward

9. This stimulates the _____ system.

renin–angiotensin–aldosterone

10. And this system (you spelled it, I'm not going to) causes retention of _____ and thus _____.

sodium water

11. So we can conclude that forward heart failure (ie, _____ _____ _____ output) and backward heart failure (ie, _____ of the _____ network) coexist.

insufficient left ventricular congestion venous

95

Clinical Manifestations of Right Heart Failure (pp. 105–106)
Review 18

Now we will consider the symptoms seen in a patient with right heart failure. Remember, now we are looking at a problem that is not just pulmonary, but systemic as well.

1. Overloading of the venous system causes (increased/decreased) venous pressure.

   increased

2. An early sign of overloading in the venous system is _____ of the neck veins.

   distention

3. To be significant, the distention must be visible when the patient is (in a flat position/sitting up).

   sitting up

4. Increased venous pressure forces fluid from the capillaries into the _____ tissues.

   subcutaneous

5. This fluid usually collects in the _____ parts of the body.

   dependent or lowest

6. Thus, it is called _____ _____.

   dependent edema

7. Peripheral edema may cause swelling of the _____ or _____.

   feet   legs

8. At bed rest, this edema may be found on the patient's _____.

   back

9. When edema is present throughout the entire body, it is called _____.

   anasarca

10. Pitting edema is graded from _____ to _____; the mildest edema (_____) is difficult to detect.

    1+   4+   1+

11. _____ _____ are the best way to detect fluid accumulation.

    Daily weights

12. Edema that collects in the pleural cavity is called _____ _____.

    pleural effusion

13. Edema in the peritoneal cavity is called _____.

    ascites

14. Suspect pleural effusion if, as you listen to a patient's lungs with a stethoscope, you note _____ or _____ breath sounds.

    diminished   absent

15. Pain or discomfort in the right upper abdomen may indicate edema of the _____, also due to venous distention.

    liver

16. Other symptoms that may accompany engorgement of the liver are _____ and _____.

    anorexia
    nausea

17. To detect an engorged liver, use the _____ _____ test.

    hepatojugular reflux

18. Apply pressure over the (left/right) upper quadrant of the abdomen.

    right

19. This applies pressure over the _____ and increases venous return to the heart.

    liver

20. A positive sign is _____ _____ distention, indicating the _____ _____ cannot accommodate the increased blood flow from the liver.

    neck vein   right
    heart

Treatment of Right Heart Failure (p. 106)

1. There are two goals in the treatment of right heart failure. The first is to improve cardiac _____ .

   output or performance

2. The second goal is to decrease the _____ and _____ retention.

   sodium   water

Improvement in Cardiac Performance
Review 20

1. Rest, the first step in the treatment program, (increases/decreases) diuresis, (increases/decreases) heart rate, and (increases/decreases) dyspnea.

   increases   decreases
   decreases

2. However, complete bedrest increases the risk of _____ so "chair rest" is more desirable.

   thromboembolism

3. The first line of drug therapy is the use of _____ _____.

    ACE inhibitors

4. Look at Table 7–1 (p. 101 in *The Manual*) and separate the drugs into venous dilators, arterial dilators, and combined action. Now see where they affect the mechanisms of Figure 7.4. Is it beginning to make sense?

5. You learned that ACE inhibitors can affect both _____ and _____, and in right heart failure reducing _____ is very beneficial.

    preload   afterload
    afterload

6. Beta-adrenergic agonists (_____ and _____) can be given IV but not orally.

    dobutamine   dopamine

7. Digitalis, while not used in acute _____ is a fundamental treatment for _____ heart failure.

    MI   right

Control of Sodium and Water Retention *(pp. 106–107)*

Review 21

1. A low-sodium diet may permit only _____ to _____ mg sodium per day. (Explaining the reasons for this diet may help your patient tolerate it better.)

    2000   3000

2. Sodium restriction is essential in order to decrease the circulating blood _____.

    volume

3. The average American diet contains about (2,000 mg/5,000 mg/10,000 mg/ 15,000 mg) of NA daily.

    10,000 mg

4. In addition to rest and sodium restrictions, _____ are important in the treatment of right heart failure.

    diuretics

5. Sodium and water excretion can be increased by the use of _____ drugs.

    diuretic

6. Diuretics should be used with _____ restriction, _____ _____, and, if needed, digitalis.

    NA   ACE inhibitors

7. Thiazide diuretics work on the _____ of the kidneys.

    tubules

8. Thiazides block reabsorption of _____ in the tubules and thus larger amounts of _____ and _____ are excreted.

    NA
    NA H_2O

9. Diuretics also increase excretion of _____.

    potassium

10. Low serum potassium is called _____.

    hypokalemia

11. Hypokalemia can increase myocardial _____.

    irritability

12. Increased myocardial irritability can lead to serious _____.

    arrhythmias

13. What signs and symptoms of hypokalemia would you watch for in any patient on a diuretic? _____

    lassitude   anorexia   confusion   decreased urinary output

14. Hypokalemic patients (low _____) are extremely sensitive to digitalis and predisposed to _____ _____.

    K
    digitalis toxicity

15. The most potent diuretics are _____ and _____ _____. (Trade names: _____ and _____.)

    furosemide   ethacrynic acid
    Lasix   Edecrin

16. Their extreme potency produces _____ and excessive _____ _____.

    hypokalemia   fluid
    loss

17. _____ replacement therapy is almost always necessary in patients on these drugs.

    Potassium

18. Patients with increased sodium loss due to diuresis and restricted sodium diets, may need to have their fluids (increased/restricted).

    restricted

19. High fluid intake under these conditions may result in _____.

    hyponatremia (low-salt syndrome)

20. Remember Figure 7–4? Angiotensin II stimulates the release of _____ from the adrenal cortex and that (increases/decreases) reabsorption of NA and water from the kidneys.

aldosterone
increases

21. Spirolactone (_____) is an aldosterone antagonist and promotes _____ of NA.

Aldactone
excretion

22. Aldosterone antagonists are (more/less) potent than thiazides and their action is slower.

less

Drug Review/Practice
Review 22

The more you learn about drugs and their actions now, the easier it will be later on. So, let's do some matching of generic and trade names. Place the correct number of the "Trade" or "brand" name in front of the generic name.

Generic	Trade	
_____ Prazosin	1. Apresoline	8
_____ Sodium nitroprusside	2. Isordil	5
_____ Captopril	3. Capoten	3
_____ Isosorbide dinitrate	4. Sorbitrate	4
_____ Isosorbide dinitrate	5. Nipride	2
_____ Hydralazine	6. Loniten	1
_____ Minoxidil	7. Regitine	6
_____ Phentolamine	8. Minipress	7

Diuretic ABC
Review 23

Match the letters, A, B, and C with the correct statements. More than one letter may be required for some statements.
  A—Thiazides
  B—Lasix or Edecrin
  C—Aldosterone antagonists

_____ 1. Highest potency	B	
_____ 2. Next highest potency	A	
_____ 3. Fastest acting	B	
_____ 4. Acts in 2 to 5 days	C	
_____ 5. Acts within 2 hours	A	
_____ 6. Blocks reabsorption of sodium in tubules	A, B	
_____ 7. Acts against the hormone that causes the body to retain salt	C	
_____ 8. Usually given as IV	B	
_____ 9. Potassium therapy nearly always required	B	
_____ 10. Aldactone is an example	C	
_____ 11. Ethacrynic acid is another name for _____	B	Edecrin
_____ 12. Hydrochlorothiazide is one example of this diuretic	A	
_____ 13. Furosemide is another name for _____	B	Lasix

Review 24

Shall we apply what you have just learned? Let's take the 3 P.M. report on Mr. Kardiak in CCU.

"Mr. Kardiak has been in normal sinus rhythm, rate around 88. At 2 P.M. his rate was 94. No arrhythmias noted. His lungs show some rales in the left posterior base. Respiratory rate 12 to 18. His neck veins are not distended. Hepatojugular reflux negative. He has seemed a little tired and lethargic today; however, the night shift reported he slept poorly, so maybe that explains it."

The day shift trots off to a ballgame or a concert, and you put away thoughts of your morning tennis game or jam making and prepare for a busy evening in CCU. Because Mr. Kardiak is doing so well, you assign him to another nurse. It's 8 P.M. before you have time to review his vital signs sheet. This is what you note:

$$4 \text{ P.M.:} \quad 99\text{—}98\text{—}18$$
$$6 \text{ P.M.:} \quad 99^2\text{—}102\text{—}20$$
$$8 \text{ P.M.:} \quad 99^2\text{—}112\text{—}26$$

Grabbing your favorite red stethoscope, you head for his bedside.

1. Before you pounce on Mr. Kardiak with your cold stethoscope, you (circle all the appropriate answers.)
   A. make small talk
   B. introduce yourself
   C. ask if he feels weak and fatigued
   D. ask how he feels
   E. ask if he feels different from yesterday or this morning
   F. explain that you want to listen to his heart and lungs

   B D E F

Answers and Comments

A. You don't have time for small talk.
C. A direct question like this plants the idea and may shape the patient's response.

Don't put words in his mouth. Ask general questions and then follow them up with more specific questions.

2. Now ask Mr. Kardiak to sit up and let's listen to

   A. his lungs for _____ and evalute _____ _____ _____.

   rales   shortness of breath

   B. his heart for _____ _____.

   gallop rhythm

   While you are listening you also note:

   C. skin in general for _____ or _____.

   cyanosis   pallor

   D. sacral area for _____.

   edema

   E. neck for _____ _____.

   distended veins

3. Finished? Let him lie back and then check the following:

   A. _____ _____ quadrant of the abdomen.

   Right upper

   B. You are checking for _____ _____.

   liver enlargement

   C. You press firmly in and up (under the rib cage) to check for _____ _____.

   hepatojugular reflux

   D. While pressing you watch the _____ _____.

   neck veins

   E. If they fill and stand out, it's a (positive/negative) sign.

   positive

   F. Which, in our way of looking at things, is (good/bad).

   bad

Now that you have finished, you have noted the following:

- Tachycardia
- A sweating, tired, lethargic patient
- Rales on both sides
- S$_3$ gallop
- Distended neck veins at a 45° sitting angle
- Positive hepatojugular reflux

Would you call the doctor away from his favorite baseball game? _____

Evaluating the Response to Therapy (pp. 108–109)
Review 25

When the crisis is over the doctor goes home, but you still have a vital role. Think about what you are looking for and why, as you consider these questions. Discussion answers follow.

1. Routine urine outputs. Routine daily weights. Is it just more routine?

2. And you have more important things to do than recording Mr. Kardiak's intake. Right?

3. What vital signs (including hemodynamic) are important. Why?

4. Examine and assess the patient carefully. Why?

5. Mr. Kardiak is on digitalis. Why would you watch his monitor closely?

6. His lab reports show hypokalemia. Why are you concerned?

Answers and Discussion

1. Improved kidney function leads to increased urinary output—a sign that therapy is working. This is no time to say, "I guess there is more urine in his Foley bag." Know down to the last cc what the output is. Further drug and IV therapy often hinges on exactly what the urine output is. Daily weights (at the same time every day) will help you detect fluid retention before it shows in other ways.

2. Overloading this patient with IV fluids is just as destructive as a heavy spring rain on a dammed-up mountain stream. On the other hand, a high or normal fluid intake can lead to hyponatremia in a patient who is on diuretics and a sodium-restricted diet. Keep an hourly tab on his intake and output, and know what kind of deficit between the two is tolerable. Call the doctor promptly when the difference between intake and output goes beyond the tolerable range.

3. Heart rate and rhythm, respirations, blood pressure, right atrial pressure, PCWP, cardiac output, S$\bar{\text{v}}$o$_2$. You are watching for arrhythmias that could be caused by drugs, hypokalemia, or hypoxia. Vasodilators can cause hypotension.

4. Your ability to detect the first negative signs and intervene may be the difference between life and death for Mr. Kardiak. And his subsequent therapy is based on your observations and assessments.

5. Digitalis can cause serious arrhythmias if the dosage is excessive. The amount of digitalis required varies with each patient. You must watch the monitor and the patient for signs of overdose (toxicity). What signs? You will study arrhythmias beginning with Chapter 10, and you will see the frequent notation, "May be caused by digitalis." The patient? Watch for nausea, vomiting, diarrhea, headaches, and the patient who says, "Something's wrong with my eyes—I see funny colors." (Green and yellow seem to be popular.)

6. Hypokalemia predisposes to arrhythmias. The poor patient! Decreased oxygenation and electrolyte imbalance can cause arrhythmias; diuretics cause hypokalemia, which causes arrhythmias. Everything is against him. He really needs an alert nurse to detect and treat these problems.

Initiating Emergency Treatment for Acute
Pulmonary Edema *(pp. 109–110)*

Review 26

Mr. Kardiak improved. Now it is several days later and suddenly he is in trouble again. He is gasping, gurgling, and coughing up bubbly, bloody mucus. He is struggling frantically for breath and is drenched with perspiration. (Check your answers below)

1. Mr. Kardiak appears to have _____ _____ _____.

2. You can do three things instantly and simultaneously.

   a. _____

   b. _____

   c. _____

3. While you are putting the oxygen mask on, try to _____ him that oxygen will help his breathing.

4. Drugs the doctor may order immediately are _____, and a rapid-acting _____.

5. You can titrate Mr. Kardiak's vasodilators according to his pulmonary artery catheter readings (unless your protocol dictates otherwise). How? _____

   _____

   _____

6. You are going to watch the monitor closely for _____ on this patient.

7. Ask the doctor if he would like to have _____ _____ _____ drawn.

8. What is the most important thing you can do for this patient and his family? _____

   _____

   _____

Answers and Comments

1. *Acute pulmonary edema.*

2. *Help the patient to a sitting position in bed, give him oxygen,* and *call the doctor.* (Obviously you need four hands or else a helper.) At this point some patients fight the oxygen mask or insist that no air is coming out of it. Reassurance, turning the oxygen up temporarily so they can feel it, letting them hold the mask—sometimes these things help.

3. *Reassure* the patient. Many patients cry, "Let me get to a window for some air!" It may help to reassure them that oxygen will do them more good and that scrambling around will only increase their air hunger.

4. *Morphine,* and a rapid-acting *diuretic.* All will probably be given IV.

5. Titrate to maintain the PCWP between 12 to 15 mm Hg and the systemic vascular resistance between 800 and 1200 dynes/sec/cm^{-5}.

6. *Arrhythmias.* There is an especially high risk of arrhythmias developing when oxygenation is inadequate.

7. *Arterial blood gases* are frequently ordered.

8. Explain. Reassure. Do it again. Mr. Kardiak is scared to death and so is his family. And you are storming around there without saying a word to anyone! You may have more than one cardiac arrest on your hands!

CARDIOGENIC SHOCK (pp. 110–115)

Review 27

Cardiogenic shock is a terrible killer. In many hospitals, at least 8 out of 10 patients with cardiogenic shock die. If we only knew for certain what causes cardiogenic shock and exactly how it progresses, perhaps we could treat it effectively. Unfortunately, we don't and we can't. Detecting the earliest signs of cardiogenic shock is currently our best approach, but it is not a real solution. However, if you are vigilant, your patient might be one of the lucky ones who survives. Our discussion begins with some familiar phrases: *inadequate perfusion, stroke volume,* and *cardiac output.*

1. When the left ventricle pumps out less blood at each stroke, there is a decrease in _____ _____.

   stroke volume

2. If stroke volume decreases markedly, _____ _____ will also decrease.

   cardiac output

3. In cardiogenic shock, cardiac output is severely _____.

   decreased

4. Let's get specific. In cardiogenic shock, cardiac output drops below _____ L/min, and systolic BP is less than _____ mm Hg.

   2.0
   90

5. Forty percent or more of the myocardium may be destroyed, thus a decreased stroke volume (increases/decreases) preload and myocardium receives (more/less) blood.

   increases   less

6. Also hypotension (increases/decreases) coronary perfusion and ischemia worsens and may turn to _____.

   decreases
   necrosis

7. The body may compensate for decreased cardiac output by constricting peripheral _____.

   arterioles

8. This peripheral vasoconstriction tends to divert more blood internally to _____ _____.

   vital
   organs

9. When perfusion is no longer adequate, _____ _____ receive inadequate blood and oxygen and it is termed _____ _____.

   vital organs
   inadequate perfusion

10. Inadequate perfusion may damage certain _____ systems.

    enzyme

11. In the last stages of cardiogenic shock, blood vessels dilate and the circulation _____.

    collapses

12. When this happens, cardiogenic shock is termed _____ shock.

    irreversible

13. With irreversible shock, _____ is inevitable.

    death

Clinical Manifestations of Cardiogenic Shock (pp. 110–112)

Do you believe you have a "sixth sense"? Well, coupled with keen nursing observation, I might believe it. Have you ever said, "I've got a funny feeling about that patient. He's restless and he seems different." Is this intuition, or are you detecting the first signs of cardiogenic shock?

Review 28

1. Decreased perfusion to the brain often causes _____ changes.

   mental

2. The first signs of this are _____ and _____.

   apathy   lassitude

3. Inadequate perfusion of the kidneys causes decreased _____ _____.

   urinary volume

4. If the urinary output falls below _____ cc/hour, be suspicious of decreased cardiac output.

   60

5. If the output decreases each hour, you should _____ _____ _____.

   tell the doctor

6. Decreased urinary output is called _____.

   oliguria

102

7. Urinary output of less than _____ cc/hour is usually a bad sign.

20

8. No output, that is, _____, is ominous.

anuria

9. In cardiogenic shock the blood pressure _____ as a result of decreased cardiac output, usually the systolic goes below _____ mm Hg.

falls
90

10. All patients with hypotension have cardiogenic shock. (True/False)

False

11. The numerical difference between systolic and diastolic blood pressure is called the _____ _____.

pulse pressure

12. In cardiogenic shock the pulse pressure is _____.

reduced

13. Because of peripheral vasoconstriction, the patient's skin becomes _____ and _____.

cold
pale

14. At the same time, stimulation of the central nervous system causes the skin to be _____ or _____.

wet   clammy

15. Normal cellular metabolism utilizing oxygen is called _____ metabolism.

aerobic

16. The end product of aerobic metabolism is _____ acid.

carbonic

17. The body excretes carbonic acid through the lungs as _____ _____.

carbon dioxide

18. In cardiogenic shock there is not enough oxygen for _____ metabolism.

aerobic

19. Therefore the body turns to _____ metabolism to preserve cellular life.

anaerobic

20. Anaerobic metabolism produces _____ acid.

lactic

21. The body can't get rid of lactic acid through the lungs or kidneys so it builds up in the _____.

blood

22. This creates a condition called _____ _____.

lactic acidosis

23. Body _____ or _____ cannot live in an acidotic environment.

cells   tissues

24. Also, in the presence of acidosis, fatal _____ may occur.

arrhythmias

25. Therefore, acidosis cannot be tolerated and _____ must be used to combat it.

alkalis

Treatment of Cardiogenic Shock (pp. 112–113)
Review 29

1. Cardiogenic shock must be treated _____ for best results.

immediately

2. There (is/is no) standardized treatment. Treatment, including drug therapy, must be based on repeated assessment of the patient's _____ status.

is no
hemodynamic

3. Mechanical assistance (_____ or _____) may be needed if other therapies are inadequate.

IABP   VAD

4. Surgical treatment, _____ _____ is the only hope for some patients.

cardiac transplant

5. Early detection and treatment are based on you (the nurse) identifying five signs and symptoms:

   1. _____

   reduced mental alertness

   2. _____

   decreased blood pressure

   3. _____

   narrowed pulse pressure

   4. _____

   decreased urinary output

   5. _____

   skin that is pale, cool, and clammy

Hemodynamic and Physiologic Measurements *(pp. 112–113)*
Review 30

1. Intra-arterial catheters (passed through _____ or _____ arteries) allow _____ BP measurement.

   radial   brachial
   direct

2. Mr. Kardiak has a pulmonary artery catheter. You measure _____ to identify any increase in _____. (Initials, please.)

   PCWP
   LVEDP

3. LVEDP is one of the earliest and most important indications of diminished _____ _____ function.

   left
   ventricular

4. Using a _____ pulmonary artery catheter allows you to measure cardiac output.

   thermodilution

5. Two important arterial blood gases are Pao$_2$ and pH; they show inadequate _____ and metabolic _____.

   oxygenation   acidosis

6. Arterial blood gases (should/should not) be performed while the patient is on oxygen.

   should

7. Pao$_2$ below _____ shows positive pressure ventilation is indicated.

   75 mm Hg

8. Pain should be relieved with (oral/IM/IV) medication.

   IV

9. Why that route? _____ _____

   Absorption decreases with poor circulation.

10. As you recall, during cardiogenic shock the body reverts to _____ metabolism because of poor perfusion.

    anaerobic

11. An end product of anaerobic metabolism is _____ _____.

    lactic acid

12. Lactic acidosis may lead to lethal cardiac _____.

    arrhythmias

13. Lactic acidosis is treated with _____ _____.

    sodium bicarbonate

14. Complete your own pH scale below. Fill in the normal pH range and insert the terms *acidosis* and *alkalosis* under the scale in the correct places (1 and 2).

    Normal pH range = _____ to _____

    7.30   7.35   7.40   7.45   7.50

    1. _____   2. _____

    7.35   7.45

    1. acidosis
    2. alkalosis

15. pH values below _____ indicate acidosis.

    7.35

Specific Treatment (Drug Therapy) *(pp. 113–114)*

Infusion of Fluids

Review 31

About 10% of the cardiogenic shock patients respond to plasma volume expansion. Identification and treatment of this small group are worthwhile. How can you identify those few patients who might respond to volume expansion?

1. When we speak of patients with a dangerously depleted circulating plasma volume, we say they are _____. (Nurses often say they are dried out like prunes, but that is not the answer!)

   hypovolemic

2. Consider the causes of this condition in a patient with severe MI: he loses fluids due to _____ and _____.

   vomiting   diaphoresis

3. Also, he is probably being treated with _____ to increase fluid output.

   diuretics

4. We are afraid of overloading a weak heart so we curtail IV intake. The patient also suffers from _____, so he eats and drinks little.

   anorexia

5. Unless we are careful we will end up with a low _____ volume.

plasma

6. PCWP on this patient would be (low/normal/high).

low or normal

7. The typical cardiogenic shock patient has (low/normal/high) PCWP readings.

high

8. With a low PCWP, plasma _____ _____ can be used to see if blood pressure and urine output increase.

volume expansion

9. In this situation, you might expect an order to administer 200 cc D_5W in _____ minutes.

10

10. In marked volume depletion, expect to use albumin, whole blood, or _____ _____.

low-molecular-weight dextran

Inotropic Drugs
Review 32

1. Inotropic drugs are used to _____ the pumping ability of the heart.

strengthen

2. Inotropic drugs also (decrease/increase) myocardial oxygen consumption.

increase

3. This effect is (dangerous/desirable).

dangerous

4. Norepinephrine (trade name: _____) and dopamine (trade name: _____) are two inotropic drugs frequently used.

Levophed   Inotropin

5. Another inotropic drug is dobutamide or trade name _____.

Dobutrex

6. During inotropic drug therapy, you would be satisfied if the patient had a systolic pressure of _____ to _____.

90   100 mm Hg

7. As the drugs are being administered, you watch the monitor for _____.

arrhythmias

8. You expect the drugs to act within (10 to 30 minutes/1 hour/3 hours).

1 hour

9. _____, the opposite of vasopressor drugs, may be tried on a limited number of patients suffering from cardiogenic shock.

Vasodilators

10. The theory of vasodilator therapy is that there is so much peripheral vasoconstriction that the left ventricle suffers because _____ _____.

it has to pump against such strong resistance

11. Thus, _____ drugs may be used to decrease peripheral resistance.

vasodilator

12. The disadvantage is that vasodilators (lower/raise) blood pressure.

lower

13. Vasodilators may be used if a patient's systolic pressure is above _____.

90 mm Hg

14. Increased systemic vascular resistance (greater than 1200 dynes/sec/cm^{-5}) is indication for the use of _____.

vasodilators

15. Two drugs that may be effective in these conditions are sodium _____ and _____.

nitroprusside
phentolamine

16. Drugs or pacing may be used to maintain a heart rate of between _____ and _____ beats/min.

60
100

Mechanical Assistance of the Circulation *(pp. 114–115)*
Review 33

Perhaps you are tired of filling in the blanks. Let's try a few straightforward questions.

1. What does the survival of the cardiogenic shock patient finally depend on (ie, what physiological basis)? _____

_____

2. Although inotropic drugs may help, they also have what serious side effects? _____

_____

3. If cardiogenic shock patients do not respond to drug therapy, what procedure should be considered next? _____

_____

Answers

1. The amount of oxygen available to the myocardium and the degree of tissue perfusion.

2. Inotropic drugs increase myocardial oxygen consumption; thus the heart requires more oxygen than before.

3. Mechanical assistance or intraaortic balloon pump (IABP).

Intraaortic Balloon Pump *(pp. 114–115)*
Review 34

1. Blood enters the coronary arteries during (systole/diastole).   diastole

2. The blood supply to the coronary arteries is from the _____.   aorta

3. An increase in aortic pressure during diastole might (decrease/increase) the filling of the coronary arteries.   increase

4. The IABP does this by inserting and inflating a balloon in the aorta at the onset of (systole/diastole).   diastole

5. The balloon catheter is inserted in the aorta through the _____ artery.   femoral

6. A pump inflates the balloon with _____ at the onset of diastole.   helium

7. The pump deflates the balloon _____ _____ _____ to decrease resistance when the heart contracts.   just before systole

8. The sudden decrease in aortic pressure (reduces/increases) the workload of the left ventricle.   reduces

9. The IABP is synchronized with (respirations/heartbeat).   heartbeat

10. It has proven very difficult to _____ patients away from IABP.   wean

Ventricular Assist Device *(p. 115)*
Review 35

1. VAD can be used for the (left ventricle/right ventricle/or both).   both

2. A _____ is placed in the right or left atria (or both for biventricular failure) and the blood routed through _____ _____.   cannula
assist pump(s)

3. Total systemic blood flow (including _____ _____ and _____ _____ _____ is maintained at 2.2 L/min/M$_2$.   ventricular output   VAD
pump flow

4. Left atrial pressure or pulmonary artery wedge pressure is maintained at _____ to _____ mm Hg by adjusting flow.   5
15

5. Most CCUs require a team in attendance consisting of a surgeon, two _____ _____, and a perfusionist.   CCU nurses

6. IABP and VAD (have/have not) made a significant impact on cardiogenic shock mortality.   have not

7. Sometimes a coronary _____ operation with a resection of _____ myocardium can be effective.   bypass   noncontractile

8. Cardiac transplant may be an option for patients who are less than _____ years of age, and have no irreversible _____ _____ or life-threatening illnesses.   65
organ damage

106

9. It is also important that transplant candidates be _____ sound and have good _____ support. | mentally
social

10. Survival rates with cardiac transplant are: one year = _____%, five years = _____%. | 90
50

PATIENT AND FAMILY EDUCATION AND COUNSELING *(pp. 115–116)*

Review 36

1. Patients and families need to understand their _____, _____, and expected outcomes. | condition   treatment

2. Realistic expectations are important but sustaining _____ may be more important. | hope

3. People under stress do not absorb instruction well so _____ instruction is necessary. | printed

Electrocardiographic Interpretation of Arrhythmias

CARDIAC ELECTRICAL SYSTEM REVIEW

Welcome to the fascinating world of monitoring! Before long, I hope monitors will become your best friend. Perhaps you have wondered why such a fuss is made over the diagnosis of arrhythmias. Simply, because arrhythmias can kill.

And why do we worry about the *type* or classification of arrhythmias we are seeing? Because different arrhythmias require different treatments. Some are dangerous; some are not dangerous. And some arrhythmias require no treatment.

Before we begin, please, let me convince you of one thing. You can't just memorize arrhythmia patterns from this or any other book. You can't look at page 125, Figure 8–12 in *The Manual* for example, and say, "That's the way all normal sinus rhythms (NSR) will look. Anything else is an arrhythmia and should be treated." None of your patients looks exactly alike physically—why should they be identical electrically?

You must take time to learn the meaning of each part of the electrical patterns and know the limits of normal. Then be familiar with the diagnostic criteria for each arrhythmia; but, please, don't try to memorize patterns. I know of no shortcuts to interpreting arrhythmias. One thing is certain: You must be able to recognize *normal* before you can diagnose *abnormal.*

We will go through this important chapter step by step, using a series of questions and answers.

Before we begin, go back to Chapter 3 and try Reviews 1, 2, and 3 again. Be sure you know that material and then we will add more detail now. (Use Fig. 8–1 in *The Manual.*)

Review 1

1. The normal cardiac pacemaker (ie, the _____ _____) normally "fires" _____ to _____ times per minute.

   SA node   60
   100

2. The electrical impulses from the SA node travels through three _____ tracts in the _____ atrium to the _____ node, down through the _____ _____ _____ where the conduction system then branches off into the _____ _____ _____ and the _____ _____ _____.

   internodal
   right   AV
   bundle of His   right bundle
   branch   left bundle branch

3. The _____ bundle branch has two divisions: the _____ _____ and the _____ _____.

   left   anterior superior
   posterior inferior

4. The final goal is to stimulate the _____ myocardial cells.

5. This causes a discharge of electrical forces stored across the _____ _____.

6. The name for this discharge is _____ and it results in cardiac _____.

7. Then the muscle cells must restore their _____ _____ and recover so they can discharge again; this period is called _____.

8. Depolarization and repolarization are the electrical events of the _____ _____.

9. The chemical process involves the exchange of _____ and _____ ions during the electrical events of the cardiac cycle.

Purkinji

cell
membranes

depolarization
contraction

electrical charge
repolarization

cardiac
cycle

Na   K

THE ELECTROCARDIOGRAM *(pp. 118–122)*

Review 2

I am sure you have watched technicians taking an ECG, and you know that they strap little electrodes on all four limbs. Then they place another electrode on the chest wall and move it from place to place. The purpose of these multiple electrodes is to get several different views of the heart's electrical activity. In fact, by simply switching a knob on the ECG machine, twelve separate views—or leads—can be obtained. This is called a 12-lead electrocardiogram. Each lead shows a different electrical pattern on the ECG, as the flow of current being recorded is from different electrode positions.

First, we will discuss the three leads called the *standard limb leads* because they are recorded from the limb electrodes. Actually, only three of the four limb electrodes are "working" electrodes. The fourth, on the right leg, is only a ground wire, so we can ignore it. Now if we take the three working electrodes—those on the right arm, left arm, and left leg— and join them in a theoretical triangle, we can see the three limb leads (Fig. 8.1.).

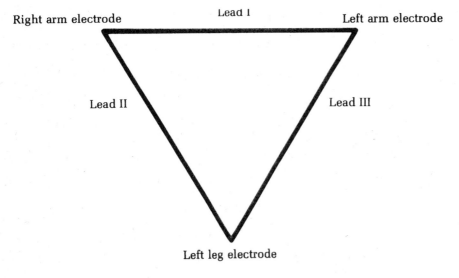

Figure 8.1

Electrocardiography Leads *(pp. 118–119)*
Review 3

1. Do leads I, II, and III make sense to you? If not, take six pieces of tape and write one of the following on one of the pieces: I+, I–, II+, II–, III+, III–.

2. Place the tapes on your arms and legs (as ECG technicians place the electrodes) or on your shoulders and thigh for convenience. Place I– on your right shoulder and I+ on

your left shoulder. Lead I records the difference in potential of depolarization coming from the right toward the left electrode.

3. Now place II– on your right shoulder and II+ on your left thigh. Again the difference in potential shows electrical forces traveling from negative (right arm) to positive (left thigh).

4. Finally place III– on your left shoulder and III+ on your left thigh. Lead III will show the electrical forces flowing from left shoulder to left thigh as a positive deflection.

Now can you "see" what the three positive limb electrodes are seeing? Look at some of the R waves in actual ECGs. The higher the R wave, the greater the difference in electrical potential sensed by the positive electrode. All negative waves were "traveling away from" the positive electrode.

Review 4

1. A lead consists of (one/two) electrodes.

two

2. One of the electrodes is a positive pole and the other a _____ pole.

negative

3. When electrical impulses flow *toward* a positive electrode, the ECG will record an upward deflection. When impulses flow *away* from a positive electrode, the deflection will be _____.

downward

4. The average of the electrical forces generated during depolarization is called the _____ _____.

electrical axis

5. If the electrical _____ goes _____ the + pole the ECG will record an upward (ie, _____) deflection.

axis   toward
positive

6. If the _____ axis goes away from the _____ pole, a downward (or _____) deflection records on the ECG.

electrical   positive
negative

7. If the _____ _____ goes perpendicular to the axis of the lead, there is _____ deflection.

electrical axis
no

8. Lead I records electrical forces flowing between the right arm electrode and the _____ arm electrode.

left

9. Leads II records electrical forces flowing between the right arm electrode and the _____ _____ electrode.

left leg

10. Leads III records the electrical forces flowing between the _____ _____ and _____ _____ electrodes.

left arm
left leg

11. In lead I, the right arm electrode is negative and the left arm electrode is _____.

positive

12. Therefore, cardiac impulses that travel in the direction of right arm to left arm will cause an (upward/downward) deflection on the ECG.

upward

13. In lead I, the normal flow of current is between the _____ arm and the _____ arm (*see* Fig. 8–2 on page 119 of *The Manual*).

right
left

14. Normally, lead I should cause an _____ deflection on the ECG.

upward

15. In lead II, the right arm electrode is negative and the left leg electrode is _____.

positive

16. Cardiac impulses flowing from the right arm toward the left leg will cause an _____ deflection on the ECG.

upward

17. This represents the normal flow of current in lead II. However, if for some reason impulses flowed *away* from the left leg (the positive electrode), the deflection would be _____.

downward

18. In lead III, either the left arm or left leg can be the positive electrode, depending on the position (or axis) of the heart. If the left leg electrode is positive, the right arm will then be _____.

negative

19. In this case, impulses from the heart traveling in the direction of left arm to left leg will cause an _____ deflection on the ECG.

upward

20. But if impulses travel in the opposite direction (from left leg to left arm), the deflection will be _____.

downward

The 12-Lead Electrocardiogram *(pp. 119–121)*
Review 5

1. The twelve leads include three standard _____ leads, three _____ leads, and six _____ leads.

limb   augmented
chest or precordial

2. A different classification lists three (bipolar/unipolar) and nine (bipolar/unipolar).

bipolar   unipolar

3. A bipolar lead measures the (actual/difference in) electrical potential between two electrodes.

difference in

4. A (bipolar/unipolar) lead shows the actual electrical potential at the electrode sites.

unipolar

5. The bipolar leads are _____.

leads I, II, and III

6. The other nine leads are _____.

unipolar

Review 6

On to the unipolar leads and measurement of *actual* (rather than the difference in) electrical potentials at electrode sites.

1. Now you need to imagine the _____ being the center of Einthoven's triangle.

heart

2. Next we assume that the electrical forces of the standard limb leads are equal to _____. (Canceling each other out is the way I think of it.)

zero

3. So if the center of our triangle has no electrical force (zero), the exploring (recording) electrode will show the (actual/difference in) electrical potential at its site.

actual

4. These unipolar electrodes (do/do not) use the same three limbs.

do

5. The unipolar voltages are very low and must be electrically _____.

augmented

6. Thus these leads are called the _____ unipolar leads.

augmented

7. They are designated aVR, (augmented _____ _____ arm); aVL, (_____ unipolar _____ arm); aVF, (augmented unipolar _____ _____).

unipolar right
augmented   left   left leg
("foot" makes better sense!)

8. That wasn't so bad, was it? Now we have only six more unipolar leads; these are recorded from the _____.

chest or precordium

9. The ECG technician (or you) moves an electrode across the _____ to record the (actual/difference in) electrical potential coming toward the electrode.

chest
actual

10. There are (3/6/9/12) chest leads.

six

11. These leads are called (c/v) leads, and they move from (left to right/right to left) (see p. 122, Fig. 8–7 in *The Manual*).

v, right to left

Review 7

1. Fill in the blanks in the diagram below:

Bipolar Leads	Unipolar Extremity Leads	Unipolar Chest Leads
_____	_____	_____
_____	_____	_____
_____	_____	_____
		_____
		_____
		_____

I	aVR	V1
II	aVL	V2
III	aVF	V3
		V4
		V5
		V6

Monitoring Leads *(pp. 121–122)*
Review 8

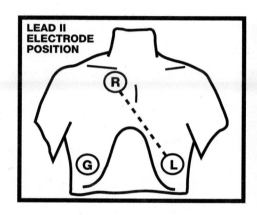 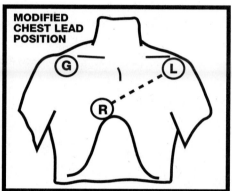

Figure 8.2

1. To review: lead II of the ECG has the positive electrode on the _____ _____ and the electrical axis of depolarization goes toward the _____ of the heart (ie, toward the left leg).

    left
    leg   apex

2. A monitor lead II gets basically the same picture because the positive electrode is placed near the _____ rib on the _____ side of the chest.

    lowest   left

3. Atrial and ventricular _____ are easily seen on lead II.

    depolarization

4. Modified chest lead I (_____) is better for monitoring ischemic changes.

    MCL_1

5. Look at Figure 8–7 in *The Manual* and locate V_1, for a 12-lead ECG. That is where you will put the positive electrode for an MCL_1.

6. The location is _____ intercostal space, _____ sternal border.

    4th   right

7. You might find _____ or _____ of these leads used in your CCU.

    either   both

ELECTROCARDIOGRAPHIC WAVE FORMS *(pp. 122–126)*

In Figure 8.3 you will see a graph with a series of little bumps, bigger bumps, and tall, narrow spikes.

Before I took my CCU course, I had patients on monitors, but I had no idea of what I was seeing or even any idea of how to describe it. One day, the ECG pattern suddenly looked very different, and in panic I called the doctor and said, "You had better come quick, there are too many little squiggles and not enough big wiggles."

Obviously, we need names for those bumps. And if you have ever tired of diagrams labeled a, b, c—take heart; for these deflections we use letters that make even less sense!

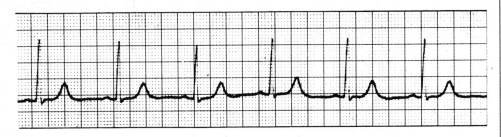

Figure 8.3

Review 9

1. The cardiac cycle involves two phases: _____ and _____.

   depolarization   repolarization

2. The ECG records the _____ _____ during the cardiac cycle.

   electrical activity

3. The electrical activity creates a series of deflections (waves) on the ECG that are labeled _____, _____, _____, _____, and _____.

   P Q R S T

4. The ECG allows us to measure the _____ of these waves.

   amplitude or voltage

5. It also allows us to measure the _____ of the waves.

   duration

ECG Measurements

ECGs are recorded on graph paper that moves through the machine at a constant speed. Without this standardized graph paper, it would be difficult to measure either the amplitude or the duration of the various waves. The graph simplifies things—if you can graph temperatures, you will be able to understand ECG measurements. So suppose we take some temps at 8 A.M., 12 noon, 4 P.M., and 8 P.M., and graph them. Now compare this graph with an ECG.

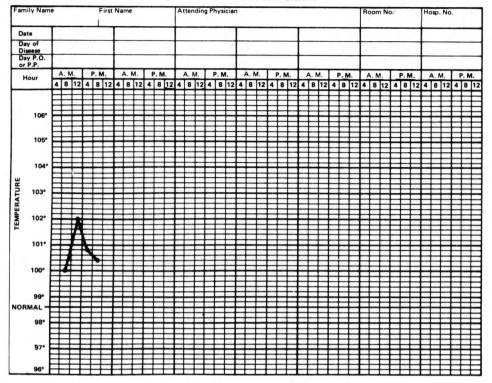

Figure 8.4. Temperature graph.

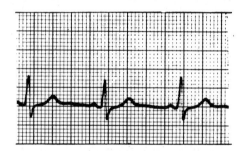

Figure 8.5. ECG

Review 10

1. Your temp graph tells you and the doctor two things: the _____ you took the temperature and the _____ of temperature.

   time
   degree or amount

2. The ECG graph also tells two things: the _____ (or duration) of an electrical impulse and the _____ of its voltage.

   time
   amount

3. Time lines on your temp graph run up and down, or _____.

   vertically

4. Similarly, time lines on the ECG run up and down, or _____.

   vertically

5. This means that the distance from one vertical line to the next vertical line on a temp graph or an ECG measures an interval of _____.

   time

6. Amount of temperature is read on lines running across, or _____ on the graph.

   horizontally

7. Amount of voltage is shown on an ECG by lines running across, or _____.

   horizontally

115

8. Thus, an ECG allows the amplitude, or _____, of an electrical wave to be measured. | voltage

9. It also shows how much _____ it took for an impulse to travel through the heart. | time

Review 11

1. If your patient's temperature goes up, the graph line goes _____. | up

2. On an ECG, an increase in voltage is shown by a line going _____. | up

3. On a temp graph, temperature is measured in units called _____. | degrees

4. On an ECG, voltage is measured in units called _____. | millivolts

5. One small square on an ECG graph (the space between two horizontal lines) equals _____ millimeter (mm). | 1

6. One millimeter represents one-tenth of a _____. | millivolt

7. How many squares high is the deflection in Figure 8.6? _____ | 10

8. This equals _____ millimeters. | 10

9. Or how many millivolts? _____ | 1 millivolt (10 × 0.1 = 1)

10. In order to save your eyesight (and sanity), you can remember that there are _____ little squares enclosed in a darker line or a big square. | 5

11. Thus, two large squares equal _____ millimeters, or _____ millivolt. | 10   1

12. The voltage of the deflection in Figure 8.7 is _____ _____ millivolts. | 1.4 millivolts (14 × 0.1 = 1.4)

13. The voltage of the deflection in Figure 8.8 is _____ _____ millivolts. | 0.6 millivolts (6 × 0.1 = 0.6)

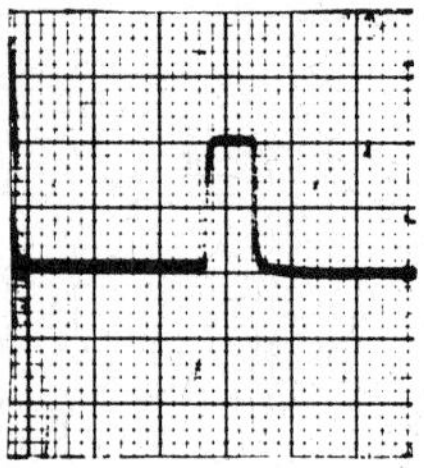

Figure 8.6 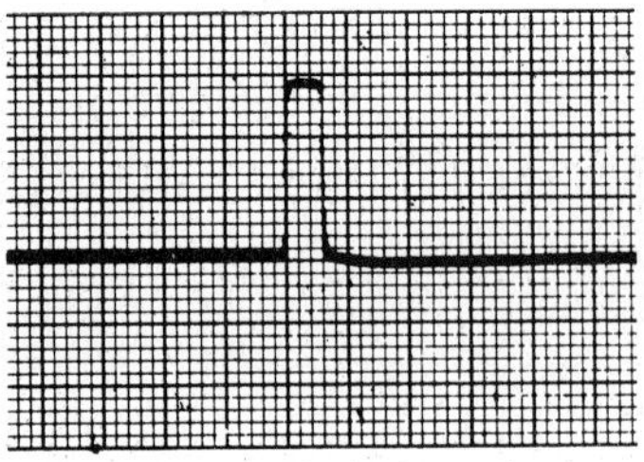   **Figure 8.7** 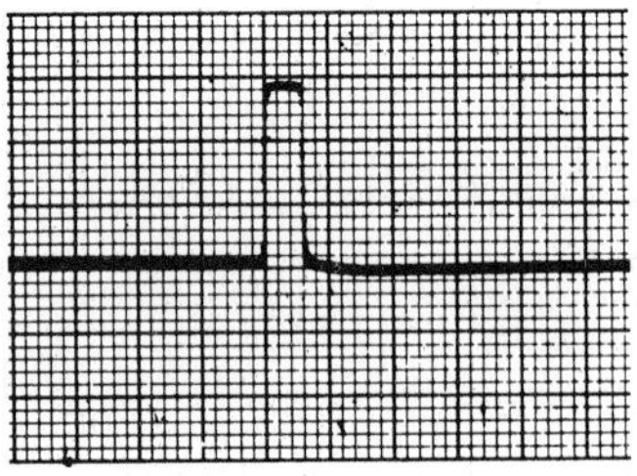   **Figure 8.8**

Review 12

You are doing fine. Now let's leave voltage and go on to time.

1. On the temp graph, time is shown in intervals of _____. | hours

2. On an ECG, time is shown in intervals of _____ of a _____. (Wow! Think about that.) | hundredths   second

3. One small square (the space between two vertical lines) equals _____ _____ seconds. | 0.04 (four hundredths)

4. Four small squares = _____ seconds. | 0.16

5. Five small squares = _____ seconds. | 0.20

6. 0.20 seconds is the same as _____ tenths of a second. (If you are weak on decimals, better review them until you are sure the above makes sense.) | two

116

7. How many small squares are enclosed in darker lines to form a larger square? _____

5

8. Five small squares = _____ seconds.

0.20

9. One large square = _____ seconds.

0.20

10. What is the duration of the deflection in Figure 8.9? _____ _____

0.24 seconds
(6 small boxes × 0.04 seconds)

11. What is the duration of the actual wave in Figure 8.10? _____ _____

0.04
(1 small box × 0.04 seconds)

12. What about the wave in Figure 8.11? (Don't let it fool you just because it's a downward (negative) wave. You count the time the same way.) _____ _____

0.16 seconds
(4 small boxes × 0.04 seconds)

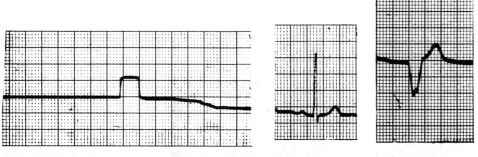

Figure 8.9   **Figure 8.10**   **Figure 8.11**

ECG Measurement Practice

If you have plodded through this far on your own, I think you are simply marvelous. Now we can proceed to put this information to practical use.

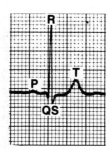

Figure 8.12. Use this ECG in answering the questions in Review 13.

Review 13

1. What is the duration of the P wave? _____ _____

about 2 small boxes or 0.08 seconds

2. What is the duration of the QRS complex? _____ _____

1 small box or 0.04 seconds

3. What is the duration of the T wave? _____ _____

about 4 small boxes or 0.16 seconds

4. What is the duration of the entire cardiac cycle (from the beginning of the P wave to the end of the T wave)? _____

        14 small boxes or 0.56 seconds

5. What is the voltage of the P wave? _____

        less than 1 small box or less than 0.1 millivolt

6. What is the voltage of the R wave? _____

        18 small boxes or 1.8 millivolts

7. Which waves have positive deflections? _____

        P, R, and T

8. Which waves have negative deflections? _____

        Q and S

The Normal Electrocardiogram *(pp. 122–128)*

You should realize that there is a wide range for normal. Just because a P wave, or any other wave, doesn't look just like the picture in a textbook, you can't say that something is wrong. Each patient's "normal" is as unique as fingerprints. You will soon develop a feel for the range of normal.

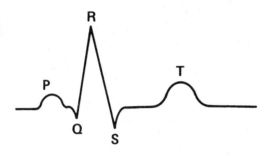

Figure 8.13. Normal cardiac cycle. (Refer to this figure in Review 14.)

Review 14

1. A normal P wave tells you that the electrical impulse started in the _____ node.

        SA

2. So, with a normal sinus pacemaker, you would see a normal _____ wave on the ECG.

        P

3. "Normal" means normal in _____ and _____.

        size   shape

4. If a P wave is not present, it means the pacemaker (is/is not) in the SA node.

        is not

5. Aberrantly shaped P waves mean that the configuration of the waves is _____

        abnormal or distorted

6. Aberrant P waves may indicate that the pacemaker (is/is not) in the SA node.

        is not

Review 15

We need to know something about the period from the beginning of the P wave to the beginning of the QRS complex, that is, the P–R interval. Try these:

1. The P–R interval is measured from the _____ of the P wave to the _____ of the QRS complex. (Just like timing a labor contraction—from the beginning of one to the beginning of the next.)

        beginning
        beginning

2. The P–R interval represents the passage of the electrical impulse from the _____ node through the _____ through the _____ node to the ventricles.

        SA
        atrium   AV

3. The normal P–R should be between _____ to _____ seconds. (Memorize the normal time limits.)

        0.12   0.20

4. A delay in the impulse passing the AV node might make the P–R (more/less) than 0.20 seconds.

more

5. If the P–R is less than .10 it shows (abnormal/normal) conduction.

abnormal

6. A shorter-than-normal (called an _____) pathway may allow the impulse to bypass the _____ node.

accessory
AV

7. These syndromes (Wolff–Parkinson–White and Lown–Ganong–Levine) are known as _____ syndromes.

pre-excitation

8. Another explanation for short P–Rs may be that the pacemaker was in the _____ node and not the _____ node.

AV   SA

9. Calculate the P–R interval in Figure 8.14. _____

0.16 seconds

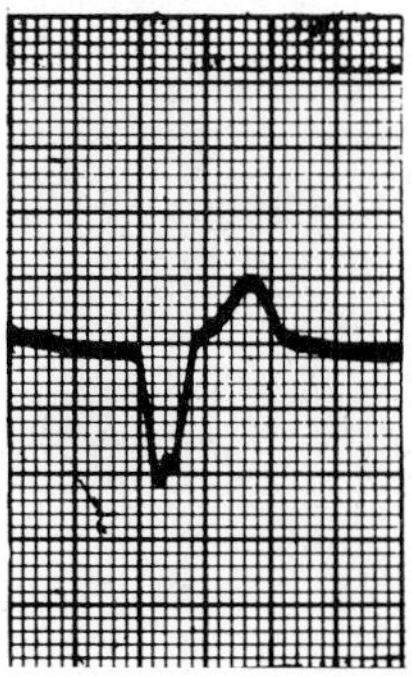

Figure 8.14

Note: If the complex (cardiac cycle) you are interpreting has a Q wave (the downward deflection), you calculate the P–R to the beginning of the Q wave. If there is no Q wave, calculate to the R wave. The Q wave is absent in some leads and hard to see in others, so don't worry about it.

Review 16

1. The QRS complex represents the depolarization of the _____.

ventricles

2. The large positive deflection is the _____ wave.

R

3. If there is a negative deflection before the R wave, it is called a _____ wave.

Q

4. Sometimes the _____ wave may be absent.

Q

5. The downward deflection after the R wave is called the _____ wave.

S

6. The total QRS should not be longer than _____ seconds.

0.12

7. In other words, it should take the electrical impulse no longer than _____ seconds to race through the ventricle.

0.12

8. Ventricular depolarization should take less than _____ seconds.

0.12

9. A QRS longer than 0.12 seconds indicates _____ conduction in the ventricles.

abnormal or delayed

Review 17

1. Depolarization of the ventricles shows in the _____ complex.

QRS

2. Repolarization of the ventricles shows in the _____ wave.

T

3. Repolarization means _____ _____

recovery or rest period after contraction.

4. The interval between the end of depolarization and the beginning of repolarization is called the _____ segment.

ST

5. The normal ST segment is (isoelectric/negative/positive). (Isoelectric means the dividing line between negative and positive. The deflection is neither upward nor downward but, rather, a straight line.)

isoelectric

6. An elevated (positive) or depressed (negative) ST may indicate muscle _____.

injury

7. An abnormal ST segment means that there is a delay in _____.

repolarization

8. One cause of this is _____

acute myocardial infarction

9. The ST segment in Figure 8.15 is (depressed/elevated/isoelectric).

depressed

10. The T wave in Figure 8.16 is _____.

inverted

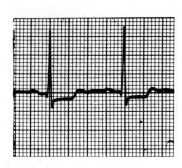

Figure 8.15

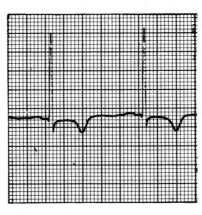

Figure 8.16

Review 18

1. The QT interval is measured from the _____ of the Q wave to the _____ of the T wave.

beginning
end

2. The QT shows the total time of _____ depolarization and repolarization.

ventricular

3. The QT duration (in normal sinus rhythm) seldom exceeds _____ seconds.

0.40

4. The QT in Figures 8.15 and 8.16 appears to be less than 0.40. (It's hard to see clearly.) This is (normal/abnormal).

normal

ECG Interpretation
Review 19

You have been working so hard, I think you deserve a treat. So let's visit a CCU. I want you to meet Nurse Dora Dom, who, poor dear, doesn't have a copy of this book. There are five patients on the monitors here, and I will run a rhythm strip of each one for you. These are not textbook pictures, but real strips from actual patients.

Now, together, let's check all 5 patients. Join in the conversation and finish what "you" starts to say.

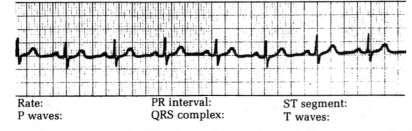

Figure 8.17
Strip 1

| Rate: | PR interval: | ST segment: |
| P waves: | QRS complex: | T waves: |

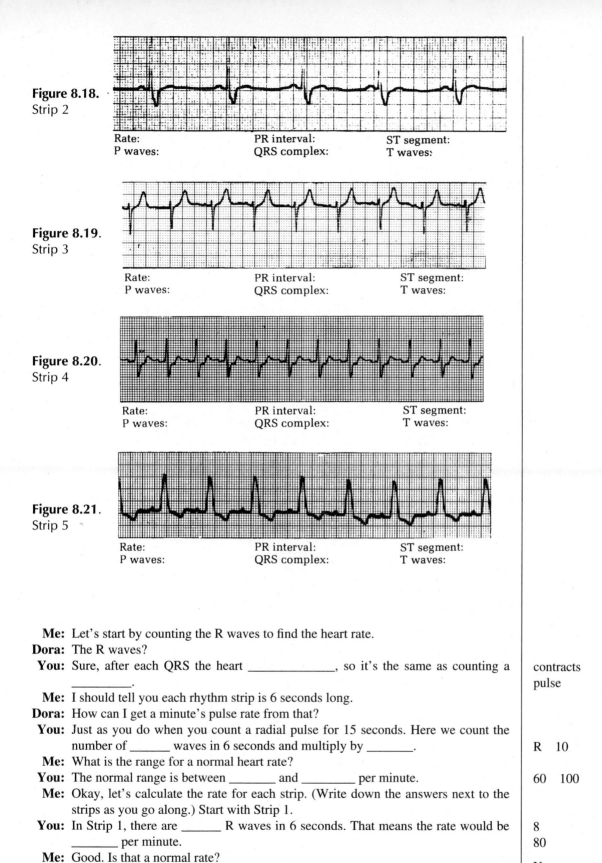

Figure 8.18.
Strip 2

Rate: PR interval: ST segment:
P waves: QRS complex: T waves:

Figure 8.19.
Strip 3

Rate: PR interval: ST segment:
P waves: QRS complex: T waves:

Figure 8.20.
Strip 4

Rate: PR interval: ST segment:
P waves: QRS complex: T waves:

Figure 8.21.
Strip 5

Rate: PR interval: ST segment:
P waves: QRS complex: T waves:

Me: Let's start by counting the R waves to find the heart rate.

Dora: The R waves?

You: Sure, after each QRS the heart _____, so it's the same as counting a _____.   contracts / pulse

Me: I should tell you each rhythm strip is 6 seconds long.

Dora: How can I get a minute's pulse rate from that?

You: Just as you do when you count a radial pulse for 15 seconds. Here we count the number of _____ waves in 6 seconds and multiply by _____.   R   10

Me: What is the range for a normal heart rate?

You: The normal range is between _____ and _____ per minute.   60   100

Me: Okay, let's calculate the rate for each strip. (Write down the answers next to the strips as you go along.) Start with Strip 1.

You: In Strip 1, there are _____ R waves in 6 seconds. That means the rate would be _____ per minute.   8 / 80

Me: Good. Is that a normal rate?

You: (Yes/No).   Yes

Me: What about Strip 2?

You: The rate is _____.   50

Me: Is that normal?

You: (Yes/No), it's below 60 per minute.   No

Me: What are slow rates called?

121

You: _____. — Bradycardia

Me: Now for Strip 3.

Dora: There's no way to count the rate in this strip—I can't see any R waves.

You: The R waves are there, all right—they are just small.

Dora: I can tell this isn't normal.

Me: How do you know?

Dora: It doesn't look like the pattern of normal in *The Manual*. I know it by heart.

Me: Not all normals look alike. You can't decide on that basis. You have to go step by step to see if anything is wrong.

Dora: Well, something's wrong with the R wave.

You: Maybe the R waves are small because of the position of the _____. — electrodes

Me: That's right. Remember what we said about how different leads give a different pattern? In this case, the R waves are small and the S waves are big because of the lead being used. Let's get back to the heart rate.

You: It's _____ per minute. — 90

Me: Normal or abnormal?

You: _____. — Normal

Me: Strip 4 is very interesting. What's the rate here?

You: It's _____ per minute. — 120

Me: Normal?

You: _____, it's greater than _____ per minute. — No 100

Me: What are fast rates called?

You: _____. — Tachycardia

Me: What's the rate in Strip 5?

You: _____ per minute, which is _____. — 80 normal

Me: Fine. You have learned a lot. Now let's analyze the P waves in each strip. Take a look at all of them and then write down whether they are normal or not.

Dora: I don't like some of them. Strips 1 and 2 seem okay, but Strip 3 is very tiny. And the shapes of Strips 4 and 5 aren't smooth and rounded.

Me: Who guaranteed that all P waves would be smooth and rounded or that they would have a certain "normal" height?

You: I think P waves in Strips _____, _____, _____, _____, and _____, are probably within normal limits. — 1 2 3 4 5

Me: Again, the configuration of the wave depends a lot on the lead being recorded. Many times you can't be sure if it's normal from a single monitor lead.

Dora: Does that mean we're through?

Me: We've only discussed rate and P waves. Now measure the P–R intervals and write down their duration.

Dora: Where do you measure from? I forgot.

You: The P–R interval is measured from the _____ of the _____ wave to the beginning of the _____ complex. — beginning P QRS

Me: What are normal values?

You: From _____ second to _____ second. — 0.12 0.20

Me: Are the P–R intervals normal in these strips?

You: _____. — Yes

Me: We are up to the QRS complex.

Dora: How do we know if the QRSs are normal? They have different shapes.

You: You measure from the _____ of the complex to the _____ of the _____. — beginning end S wave

Dora: Suppose there is no Q or S wave, then what do you do?

You: You measure the _____. — R wave

Me: What is the normal duration of the QRS?

You: It should be less than _____ second. — 0.12

Me: Measure each QRS and write down your answers. Are they all normal?

You: _____. In Strips _____ and _____ the QRSs are _____. — No 2 5 prolonged

Me: What does that mean?

You: There is some delay in _____ _____. — ventricular conduction

Me: Good thinking.

Dora: I think you missed one. In Strip 3 the QRS is only one small box or 0.04 second, as far as I can see. So there is something wrong with that one, too.

You: Nothing's wrong with the R wave, but you didn't include the _____ wave in your measurement. | S

Me: You have to measure the entire QRS complex.

Dora: Does the QRS show depolarization or repolarization of the muscle? I never can remember the difference.

You: It means _____. | depolarization

Me: Now let's look at the ST segments.

Dora: I don't remember learning a time interval for the ST segment.

Me: You're right. We didn't learn one. We are interested in the position of the segment rather than its duration. It's very important.

You: I remember—the normal ST should not be negative or positive, it should be _____. | isoelectric

Me: Very good. If it's elevated or depressed, that's a sign of injury. What causes that?

You: One cause is _____ _____. | myocardial infarction

Me: So far, so good. Now, let's go over the ST segments. Lay a piece of paper across the baseline and see if the ST segment is above or below the baseline. In other words, is the segment elevated, depressed, or isoelectric? Write down your answers for each strip.

Dora: Strip 1 is okay.

Me: What did you write down about the others? Are they normal?

You: _____. The ST segments are _____ in Strips _____. | No   depressed   4 and 5

Me: We are finally up to the T wave. Look at the T wave in the 5 strips.

Dora: They all look different. I don't understand that.

Me: There are many things that affect the T waves, and you can't expect them to look alike in each patient. We are interested mostly in whether the T waves are upright or inverted.

Dora: Why do we care about that?

You: Inverted T waves may be a sign of myocardial _____. | ischemia

Me: Right. But don't forget there are other causes as well. Now describe whether the T waves on the 5 strips are inverted or upright.

You: _____ | They are inverted in Strip 5 and upright in all the others.

Me: Were your answers right? Good. Let's celebrate! You've really got it!

Dora: *Celebrate?* Does that mean look at more ECGs?

SIGNIFICANCE OF THE ELECTROCARDIOGRAM *(pp. 127–128)*

Review 20

For variety's sake let's try some true and false questions. Complete *all* the questions before you check the answers.

1. People with normal ECGs can be assured that their immediate futures will be free from heart attacks. _____ | False

2. Coronary atherosclerosis can be diagnosed early by ECG changes. _____ | False

3. Ventricular systole (contraction) is shown on the ECG. _____ | False

4. Myocardial ischemia can be recognized on the ECG. _____ | True

5. The ECG shows only electrical activity. _____ | True

6. The ECG clearly demonstrates the physical status of the heart. _____ | False

7. The results of necrosis from previous MIs can be seen on an ECG. _____ | True

8. Ventricular systole begins with the peak of the QRS. _____ | True

9. Ventricular diastole coincides with the end of the T to the next R. _____ | True

10. The ECG shows both electrical and mechanical activity. _____ | False

Review 21

1. Technically, the word *arrhythmia* means _____ of normal rhythm.

    absence

2. In practice, however, we often mean any disturbance of _____, _____, or _____.

    rate   rhythm
    conduction

3. *The Manual* explains that arrhythmias are due to disturbances of _____ formation and disturbances of _____.

    impulse
    conduction

4. Normally, impulses are initiated by the _____ _____.

    SA node

5. Other sites where impulses can originate include the _____, _____ nodal area, and _____.

    atria   AV
    ventricles

6. Thus, one way of classifying those arrhythmias caused by disturbances of impulse formation is by the _____ of origin.

    site

7. Further classification of arrhythmias caused by disturbances of impulse formation is by the _____ of the disturbance.

    mechanism

8. If the arrhythmia has an abnormally fast rate, it is called a _____.

    tachycardia

9. If the arrhythmia has an abnormally slow rate, it is called a _____.

    bradycardia

10. The mechanism can involve some impulses coming sooner than normal. These are called _____ beats.

    premature

11. Two extremely rapid mechanisms of impulse formation are _____ and _____. These can originate either in the atria or in the ventricles.

    flutter
    fibrillation

12. Classification of arrhythmias due to conduction disturbances refers to _____ or _____ in the passage of the impulses.

    blocks
    delays

13. Conduction disturbance blocks can occur anywhere from the _____ node clear through to the _____.

    SA
    ventricles

14. However, blocks are classified according to three main sites (from the top of the heart down):

    A. Blocks *within* the _____ node and _____.

    SA   atria

    B. Blocks *between* the _____ and _____.

    atria   ventricles

    C. Blocks *within* the _____.

    ventricles

15. If we classify arrhythmias according to their seriousness, the most dangerous are labeled _____ arrhythmias.

    lethal

16. The least serious arrhythmias are called _____ arrhythmias.

    minor

17. In between these two groups is a third group of arrhythmias that are dangerous and require prompt treatment but are not immediately lethal. These are called _____ arrhythmias.

    major

Interpretation of Arrhythmias from the Electrocardiogram *(p. 129)*
Review 22

Use the five steps listed here to interpret the following ECG. Don't worry about the actual diagnosis; you will learn that later on. For now, be happy you understand the procedure involved in establishing a diagnosis. That is really progress.

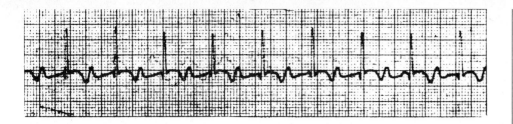

Figure 8.22

STEP 1. Calculate the Heart Rate

1. There are _____ R waves in this 6-second strip.

9

2. This means the rate is _____ beats per minute.

90

3. Is this a normal rate? _____

Yes

STEP 2. Determine the Regularity (Rhythm) of the R Waves

1. Are the R–R intervals regular? _____

Yes

2. This means the ventricular rhythm can be classified as _____.

regular

STEP 3. Identify and Examine the P Waves

1. Are they of normal size and shape? _____

Yes

2. This means the pacemaker is in the _____ _____.

SA node

STEP 4. Measure the P–R Interval

1. What is the duration of the P–R interval? _____ _____

0.32 seconds
(8 squares × 0.04 seconds)

2. Is this normal? _____

No

3. It means that there is a _____ in conduction.

delay

4. At what site? Between the _____ and _____.

atria   ventricles

STEP 5. Measure the Duration of the QRS Complexes

1. What is its duration? _____

0.10 seconds

2. Is this normal? _____

Yes

Now what have we learned from this strip?

1. The pacemaker is in the _____ _____.

SA node

2. There is normal _____ rhythm.

sinus

3. The P–R interval is _____, indicating a _____ delay between the _____ and _____.

prolonged   conduction
atria   ventricles

4. Conduction through the ventricles, however, is _____.

normal

5. How do you know this? _____ _____

The QRS duration is normal (0.10 seconds).

6. What is the site of this conduction defect? _____ _____

AV node

7. Incidentally, the T waves are _____.

inverted

8. This may indicate _____ _____.

myocardial ischemia

Review 23

Complete the statements that follow the Word Rounds. If you wish to play Word Rounds, then locate your answer in the scrambled letters. Words are spelled from left to right and downward; there is one diagonal word. Circle your words.

```
Q  B  V  E  R  T  I  C  A  L  C  S  K  G  V  C  U  D  A
E  L  E  C  T  R  O  C  A  R  D  I  O  G  R  A  P  H  T
I  L  P  V  O  L  T  A  G  E  O  N  R  I  A  M  W  Z  R
N  V  E  J  G  Z  A  R  L  C  W  U  I  E  T  P  A  B  I
T  B  C  C  E  A  S  I  N  O  N  S  G  Z  E  L  R  F  O
H  U  G  O  T  V  A  D  M  V  W  S  I  T  E  I  D  G  V
O  N  E  F  L  R  N  R  P  E  A  P  N  E  K  T  Z  K  E
V  D  V  D  Z  S  O  V  E  R  R  D  V  N  R  U  V  L  N
E  L  K  L  R  A  D  C  Z  Y  D  P  H  N  O  D  E  R  T
N  E  V  P  A  C  E  M  A  K  E  R  Z  K  L  E  N  S  R
R  Z  J  O  T  B  A  R  K  R  H  Y  T  H  M  D  Z  I  I
G  D  Q  S  E  L  V  K  V  J  D  U  R  A  T  I  O  N  C
H  O  R  I  Z  O  N  T  A  L  T  I  A  J  V  T  B  O  U
S  V  S  T  K  Z  S  L  N  L  Z  D  O  A  T  R  I  A  L
E  B  O  I  N  J  U  R  Y  V  J  E  K  G  Y  V  S  T  A
C  U  R  V  E  D  Z  J  S  T  U  L  J  E  R  D  I  R  R
O  K  V  E  L  T  A  C  H  Y  C  A  R  D  I  A  V  I  O
N  E  G  A  T  I  V  E  L  Z  D  Y  L  K  A  V  M  A  N
D  E  P  O  L  A  R  I  Z  A  T  I  O  N  B  D  C  L  E
```

Figure 8.23. Word Rounds.

1. The instrument that detects electrical waves from the heart: _____.   electrocardiograph

2. Normal cardiac pacemaker: _____ node.   sinus

3. Positive deflection on ECG: _____.   upward

4. Small lines on ECG are _____ mm apart.   one

5. Voltage: _____.   amplitude

6. Arrhythmias due to disturbances of impulse formation may be classified by the sites of _____.   origin

7. Repolarization: _____.   recovery

8. Normal cardiac pacemaker (two words): _____ _____.   SA node

9. The _____ where an arrhythmia began helps classify it.   site

10. "Battery" that discharges to cause heartbeat: _____.   pacemaker

11. The printed record of electrical waves from the heart: _____.   electrocardiogram

12. "Father of the electrocardiograph": _____.   Einthoven

13. The _____ of His conducts the impulses from the AV node to the Purkinje fibers.   Bundle

14. 10 mm = _____ mv (on ECG).

15. The distance between _____ lines measures voltage on ECG.

16. Arrhythmias originating outside the SA node but above the AV node are called _____ arrhythmias.

17. Normal P–R should not be _____ 0.20 second (one word).

18. Heart rate over 100 per minute: _____.

19. Elevated or depressed ST segments may indicate muscle _____.

20. Conduction _____ in the AV node prolongs the P–R interval.

21. Downward deflection on ECG: _____.

22. Conduction of impulse through heart: _____.

23. Another name for sinus node: _____-atrial.

24. When impulses flow away from a positive electrode, the deflection on an ECG is _____.

25. Bradycardia is a slow _____ arrhythmia.

26. Amount of time measured from one _____ line to the next = 0.04 second (on ECG).

27. Time is measured on an ECG in fractions of a _____.

28. Intensity of electrical activity of the heart: _____.

29. By counting R waves, you can calculate heart _____.

30. Island of specialized tissue in the conduction system of the heart: _____.

31. R waves in 6 seconds multiplied by _____ tells the minute rate.

32. Amount of time required for conduction: _____.

33. Normal Ps and Ts are _____ rather than pointed.

34. _____ body who can read a temperature graph can learn to read an ECG.

35. Regularity of heartbeat: _____.

The following abbreviations are also found in the Word Rounds:

1. Electrocardiogram, Anglicized: _____.

2. Electrocardiogram, German: _____.

3. Modified unipolar extremity lead (one of the twelve leads on an ECG): _____.

4. Rhythm all CCU nurses love: _____.

5. Segment on ECG that may change with injury to heart muscle: _____.

6. Normal is 0.12 to 0.20 second: _____.

7. From one R wave to the next R wave: _____.

8. Node that has a slower inherent pacing rate than SA node: _____.

one

horizontal

atrial

over

tachycardia

injury

delay

negative

depolarization

sino

downward

rate

vertical

second

voltage

rate

node

ten

duration

curved

Any

rhythm

ECG

EKG

AVR

NSR

ST

PR

RR

AV

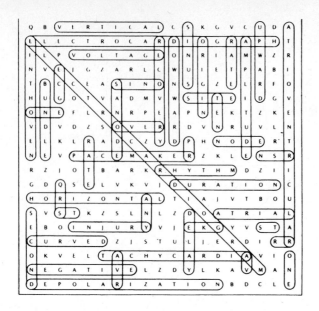

Figure 8.24. Answers to Word Rounds.

9

Arrhythmias Originating
in the Sinoatrial Node

You have arrived! You are beginning to interpret arrhythmias. I hope you are excited and enthusiastic. First, perhaps we had better get oriented; we are going to start at the top of the heart and work down. In other words, we will start at the beginning of the conduction system (the SA node) and study arrhythmias that arise there. Then we will work downward to the atria, the AV node, and the ventricles. In general, the severity of arrhythmias increases as we descend. You will soon see what I mean.

Review 1

1. You already know that the normal pacemaker is the _____ _____.

   SA node

2. Normal sinus rate is _____ to _____ beats per minute.

   60   100

3. However, the SA node can discharge _____ or _____ than 60 to 100.

   faster   slower

4. The SA node's rate is affected by the _____ and _____ nervous systems.

   sympathetic   parasympathetic

5. Increased sympathetic stimulation (speeds/slows) the heart.

   speeds

6. Increased parasympathetic stimulation (speeds/slows) the heart.

   slows

7. The electrical discharge of the SA node is shown by the _____ wave on an ECG.

   P

8. If the sympathetic and parasympathetic control become unbalanced, you may see variations in _____, _____, or _____ of impulse formation.

   rate   rhythm   site

9. A normal variation of sinus rhythm, termed _____ _____, is caused by respiration.

   sinus arrhythmia

10. Check your own pulse and correlate it with your breathing. Does your pulse increase with inspiration and decrease with expiration? If so, you have _____ _____.

    sinus
    arrhythmia

11. It is a (dangerous/warning/normal) rhythm.

    normal

12. Sick sinus syndrome may result from _____ damage to the SA node from _____ or coronary _____.

    ischemic
    AMI   atherosclerosis

13. Then the output from the SA node will vary greatly in _____.

    rate

14. As a general rule, SA node disorders are (rare/frequent) and (are/are not) dangerous.

    rare   are not

SINUS TACHYCARDIA *(pp. 136–138)*

Review 2

1. With sinus tachycardia, the pacemaker is the _____ _____.

    SA node

2. The rate is usually between _____ and _____ beats per minute.

    100   150

3. Increased stimulation of the SA node by the _____ nervous system is usually the cause of this arrhythmia.

    sympathetic

4. This overactivity is usually a reaction to _____, _____, or _____.

    fever anxiety
    activity

5. If after running around the block your pulse is 120/minute, you probably have _____ _____.

    sinus tachycardia

6. Sinus tachycardia usually terminates (suddenly/gradually).

    gradually

7. This (is/is not) a dangerous arrhythmia in its own right.

    is not

8. The danger lies in the _____ _____ of the arrhythmia.

    underlying cause

9. If it is due to fever, it may be treated with _____.

    aspirin

10. If caused by anxiety, it may be treated with _____ _____.

    relaxation techniques

11. A nurse who recognizes the faces of fear may be able to help by giving the patient _____ or _____ support.

    psychological emotional

12. The most serious cause of sinus tachycardia is _____ _____ _____.

    left ventricular
      failure

13. Chest pain from unstable _____ or an evolving _____ can cause tachycardia and should be treated immediately, usually with _____.

    angina AMI
    morphine

14. Hyperthyroidism can cause tachycardia and should be treated immediately, usually with _____.

    surgery

15. Remember the equation: stroke volume × heart rate = cardiac output? If stroke volume is reduced (due to heart failure), the heart may (increase/decrease) its rate in an attempt to maintain good cardiac _____.

    increase
    output

16. However, the increased rate (ie, tachycardia) _____ the heart's work and _____ its oxygen consumption.

    increases
    increases

17. This can lead to further heart failure, _____, and _____.

    ischemia necrosis

SINUS BRADYCARDIA *(pp. 139–141)*

Review 3

1. The pacemaker is the _____ _____.

    SA node

2. The rate is usually between _____ and _____.

    40 60

3. Increased stimulation by the _____ nervous system is often the cause.

    parasympathetic

4. Or, a phrase you will hear many times: Excess _____ stimulation slows the SA node.

    vagal

5. The rate is slow, but each normal QRS is preceded by a normal _____.

    P wave

6. Be aware that well-trained _____ or _____ people may have slower heart rates.   athletes   elderly

7. Also patients with _____ (eg, after coronary revascularization surgery) or patients with (hyperthyroidism/hypothyroidism) will have sinus bradycardia.   hypothermia / hypothyroidism

8. Some of the drugs you are giving (eg, beta _____ and _____) can cause sinus bradycardia.   blockers   verapamil

9. Verapamil is a _____ _____ _____.   calcium channel blocker

   Calcium channel blockers inhibit calcium's entrance into cells. This decreases cell contractility, dilates vessels, decreases BP, decreases peripheral resistance, decreases afterload, and decreases oxygen consumption.)

10. Think about the coronary arteries and the sites of infarctions. Most likely to cause ischemia of the SA node and thus sinus bradycardia is acute inferior MI or acute anterior MI?   acute anterior MI

11. If the sinus node _____ to below 60 per minute, other cells (ectopic foci) may pace the heart.   slows

12. Ectopic arrhythmias, especially ventricular, (are/are not) dangerous.   are

13. A significant decrease in heart rate can cause a _____ in cardiac output.   decrease

14. Severely decreased cardiac output reduces the blood supply to the _____ and arteries of the _____.   brain / heart

15. Sinus bradycardia should be considered a (lethal/warning/benign) arrhythmia.   warning

16. Uncomplicated sinus bradycardia will probably (be/not be) treated.   not be

17. Sinus bradycardia is usually treated only if it causes _____ or _____.   symptoms / complications

18. Can you list the three indications for treatment of sinus bradycardia?
    1. _____.
    2. _____.
    3. _____.
         If ventricular ectopic beats occur / If cardiac output falls / If the heart rate is less than 50

19. If the doctor does treat this arrhythmia, he will probably try _____ first.   atropine

20. Dosage will probably be _____ to _____.   0.5   1.0 mg

21. Mode of administration will be _____.   intravenously

22. Atropine blocks the _____ effect on the SA node, _____ AV conduction time, and _____ heart rate.   vagal   decreases / increases

23. If drug treatments fail and symptoms are severe, _____ _____ may be tried to speed the heart rate.   transvenous / pacing

24. Can you list some drugs you might "hold" while you call the doctor if your patient develops bradycardia? _____, _____, _____, _____.   Reserpine   digitalis / morphine   beta blockers

25. If the heart rate is less than 60 per minute, you can assume sinus bradycardia is present. (True/False)   False

26. All sinus rhythms must have a _____ wave preceding every normal QRS.   P

27. So you would check the ECG carefully for _____ waves. (No P waves? This bradycardia is not sinus. It could be more dangerous: notify the doctor.)   P

28. If the heart rate falls below _____ per minute, give atropine per protocol.   50

29. Suppose atropine is given. You would watch the heart _____ carefully to see if it speeds up.   rate

SICK SINUS SYNDROME (p. 142)

Review 4

Do you suppose they ran out of fancy names when they came to this arrhythmia? Be thankful! They could have called it atrial tachyarrhythmia-sinus bradycardia syndrome!

1. This is a rhythm of alternating _____ and _____ rates.

   fast   slow

2. How do you know it isn't sinus arrhythmia? _____ _____

   It doesn't cycle with respirations.

3. It is caused by _____ of the SA node.

   ischemia

4. A rapid _____ rhythm (eg, _____ fibrillation or _____ flutter), causes an (irregular/regular) tachyarrhythmia. (Love that new word, it just means a fast arrhythmia. Also, don't worry about the fibrillation and flutter, you will learn much more about them soon.)

   atrial   atrial   atrial   irregular

5. The slow part of the cycle is a _____ bradycardia.

   sinus

6. Sick sinus generally occurs in _____ patients.

   elderly

7. The bradycardic periods could cause a reduction in _____ and _____ blood flow.

   cerebral   cardiac

8. In a patient with heart _____ or an evolving _____, this could be serious.

   failure   MI

9. _____ may drop and the patient complain of _____.

   BP   dizziness

10. Run a strip of both _____ and _____ and also make certain you are not seeing _____ _____.

    tachycardia   bradycardia   sinus arrhythmia

11. Treatment may be a combination of _____ therapy for the tachyarrhythmia and a _____ for the bradycardia.

    drug   pacemaker

12. Initially, you would treat the bradycardia with IV _____.

    atropine

13. If the ischemia of the SA node is transient, a _____ pacemaker may be used.

    temporary

WANDERING PACEMAKER (pp. 143–145)

Review 5

1. The pacemaker may wander within the _____ node.

   SA

2. Or the pacemaker may wander away from the _____ node.

   SA

3. It may wander to the _____ _____.

   junctional area

4. The only means of diagnosis is by _____.

   ECG

5. The only ECG evidence is a change in the configuration of the _____ waves.

   P

6. This (is/is not) a dangerous or a warning arrhythmia.

   is not

7. Treatment (is/is not) required.

   is not

8. But you should watch the monitor to be sure that the _____ foci do not assume full control.

   ectopic

9. This arrhythmia probably results from increased _____ influence.

   vagal

Review 6

"Hey, Nurse, my heart just skipped a beat." The monitor gives you the information, too—a missing PQRS and T. It is not a serious problem unless the "skipping" is frequent or consecutive—then watch out!

1. The terms *sinus arrest* and *sinus block* are generally used interchangeably. (True/False)

   True

2. In sinus arrest, the sinus node _____ to fire an impulse.

   fails

3. Or the impulse is _____ within the SA node (sinus block).

   blocked

4. In either case, would you see a P wave for that interval? _____

   no

5. Would you see a QRS wave for that interval? _____

   no

6. The ECG shows no _____ _____ for one beat.

   PQRST complex

7. The usual cause is (decreased/increased) vagal influence.

   increased

8. _____ or _____ toxicity may cause sinus arrest.

   Digitalis   quinidine

9. A more dangerous cause may be _____ of the SA node.

   ischemia

10. Repeated or consecutive dropped beats can lead to _____ cardiac output.

    decreased

11. Symptoms of decreased cardiac output you should watch for are _____, _____, _____, and _____ _____.

    hypotension syncope   angina   heart failure

Review 7

Let's say your patient, Mr. Kardiak, is having sinus arrest for one beat a few times an hour.

1. On the monitor, you would note a _____ complex.

   missing

2. You had better _____ the arrhythmia on a rhythm strip.

   document (or record)

3. You would watch the monitor to see if the frequency of these missed beats _____.

   increases

4. Now it's time for Mr. Kardiak to have his digitalis. What do you do? _____ _____ _____.

   Hold the digitalis and ask if the doctor wants it given

5. You notice that the periods of sinus arrest are becoming more frequent. The doctor will probably order _____. Dosage? _____ to _____ _____.

   atropine   0.5   1 mg   IV

6. If this doesn't work _____ may be tried.

   Isuprel

7. If drug therapy doesn't work _____ _____ may be necessary.

   transvenous pacing

8. Frequent sinus arrest is a (serious-warning/lethal) arrhythmia.

   serious-warning

CHAPTER 9 REVIEW

We have covered five different types of arrhythmias so far. By now you should know how to identify them, what their dangers are, how to treat them, and what to do when they develop. Let's see how you have progressed.

Review 8

I have prepared a list of short statements that relate to one *or more* of the arrhythmias. Match the statements with the five arrhythmias. Some are easy, but others will challenge you. We will give each of the arrhythmias a letter to simplify things.

A. Sinus Tachycardia	**D.** SA Block
B. Sinus Bradycardia	**E.** Wandering Pacemaker
C. Sick Sinus	**F.** Sinus Arrhythmia

_____	1. One full cardiac cycle is missing	D
_____	2. AV node may take over	B, D
_____	3. Hold digitalis	B, D
_____	4. Cyclic pattern	C
_____	5. Digitalis may help	A
_____	6. May result from morphine	B
_____	7. Alternating fast (irregular) and slow	C
_____	8. Abnormal P waves, normal QRSs	E
_____	9. Rate increases with inspiration	F
_____	10. May be due to fever	A
_____	11. Stops gradually	A
_____	12. Patient may feel faint	C, D
_____	13. Not dangerous at all	F
_____	14. May require atropine	B, D, E, C
_____	15. Rate changes with breath holding	F
_____	16. P waves vary in configuration	E
_____	17. May be due to vagal overactivity	B, D, E
_____	18. May cause reduction in cardiac output	B, D, C
_____	19. Potentially dangerous if frequent	D
_____	20. PQRST missing	D
_____	21. May require cardiac pacing	B, D, C
_____	22. Dropped beat	D
_____	23. Rate decreases with expiration	F
_____	24. May be due to left ventricular failure	A
_____	25. Never produces symptoms	F
_____	26. Hold quinidine	B, D
_____	27. Ectopic pacemaker may take over	B, D, E, C
_____	28. Suspect calcium channel and beta blockers	B
_____	29. Aberrant P waves	E

Congratulations! You are doing excellent work.

MONITOR PRACTICE

Review 9

Let's take a look at some patients on the monitors. Fill in the blanks and answer the questions.

Patient: *Mr. Big Builder*
Diagnosis: Acute MI

Mr. BB's brother and partner in the electrical contracting business visits him. They discuss their heavy workload and contracts they may lose while BB is hospitalized. The high rate alarm rings on BB's monitor, and you see the following pattern on his scope.

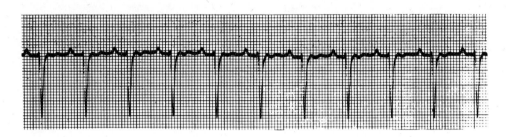

Figure 9.1

1. Arrhythmia diagnosis: _____ _____   sinus tachycardia

2. Probable cause: _____ nervous system stimulation due to _____.   sympathetic   anxiety

3. What nursing action would you take in this situation?   A, possibly B and C

    A. Call partner out of room and explain his talk is upsetting BB

    B. Tell partner visiting time is up, and he must leave.

    C. Give BB his prn tranquilizer.

    D. Tell BB he needs to relax and stop worrying.

    Think out the pros and cons of each of these choices, then read the discussion that follows.

Discussion of Nursing Action

A. Partner may not understand or cooperate; however, with some visitors it may work. Partner may then put on an act of "everything is fine." BB knows better and will worry more. BB may be upset and suspicious because you called his visitor out. How well do you know your patient and his visitors? Could you handle him this way?

B. If this isn't true, both BB and his partner will know it. If true, it should be done tactfully and courteously. BB may continue to worry and imagine worse problems than actually exist.

C. He may make a determined effort to resist the tranquilizer's effect in order to continue his business.

D. Ineffective. If he could relax, he would.

   Correct nursing action may be a combination of A, possibly B and C. It depends on your knowledge of Mr. BB. After the partner leaves, give BB a chance to talk while you give him a back rub and the tranquilizer takes effect. Two phrases you might use: "Do you want to talk about it?" and "It must be tough to . . ."

Review 10

Patient: *Mr. Kardiak*
Diagnosis: Acute MI

This man had an MI about 20 hours ago. He has taken reserpine for hypertension for six months. In the hospital the orders also include morphine every four hours, prn, potassium two times a day, and digitalis once a day. You note the following ECG on his monitor.

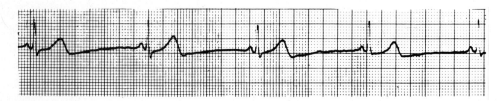

Figure 9.2

1. Arrhythmia diagnosis: _____ _____

2. Probable cause: parasympathetic nervous system (_____) dominance of the _____ _____.

3. Should you withhold drugs ordered? (Yes/No)

   If so, which drugs? _____, _____, _____

4. Notify doctor? (Yes/No)

5. Which drug would you have ready for possible treatment? _____.

6. What other treatment might be needed if rate remains too slow? _____ _____

7. Would you administer morphine if he complained of chest pain? (Yes/No)

8. The most likely treatment for this arrhythmia would be: _____

   _____
   (drug)   (dose)   (mode of administration)

sinus bradycardia

vagal   SA node

Yes

Reserpine   morphine   digitalis

Yes

Atropine

Transvenous pacing

NO, don't administer morphine.

The doctor would probably first try atropine, 0.5 to 1.0 mg, IV.

10

Arrhythmias Originating in the Atria

Now things get a bit more complicated, and I would like to try a little "tea party" to simplify them. Suppose we compare the pacemaker cells of the heart's conduction system to a group of ladies at an afternoon tea. Mrs. SA Node, who talks the fastest, usually dominates the conversation. She is the normal pacesetter. However, if she tires and slows down, her sister-in-law, Mrs. Junctional, takes over. If all the others run down, slow-speaking Mrs. Ventricle may control the conversation. Then, too, one of the slower ladies can suddenly become fired up over a topic and dominate the conversation.

Thus, the various pacemaker cells of the conduction system have the potential to take over as pacemaker for the heart under certain conditions. Or, failing to assume control, they can still impose themselves and interfere with regular rhythm. Pacemakers from ectopic foci (abnormal sites) are a possibility any time the basic rate of the heart becomes too slow.

Review 1

1. You know that the _____ _____ is the normal pacemaker of the heart.

    SA node

2. This is because it normally discharges at a (faster/slower) rate than any other area of the heart.

    faster

3. Is it possible for the SA node to be depressed and fire slower than usual? _____

    yes

4. Is it possible for an ectopic focus to become irritable and fire faster than the SA node? _____

    yes

5. What happens then? _____.

    The ectopic focus can take over

6. If the ectopic focus (or foci) is in the atria, an _____ arrhythmia develops.

    atrial

7. Atrial ectopic foci can take over for only _____ beat, or they can take over _____.

    one
    continuously

8. If atrial impulses occur at rates of less than 200 per minute, P waves can usually be seen. (True/False)

    True

9. However, the P waves are usually _____ in shape, because the pacemaker is not in the _____ _____.

    distorted
    SA node

137

Review 2

Remember, it's the atria that are contracting at fantastically rapid rates; the ventricles can't contract that fast and still manage to fill and pump out blood. So the AV node protects the ventricles from what could be serious rapidity. Now try these:

1. With very fast atrial rates, the AV node protects the ventricles by _____ some of the atrial impulses.

blocking

2. With atrial rates under 200 per minute, the AV node usually (does/does not) block atrial impulses.

does not

3. Thus, each P wave would be followed by a _____.

QRS

4. With atrial rates of 200 to 400, the AV node may _____ some, but not all, of the atrial impulses.

block

5. Thus, there will be (more/fewer) P waves than QRS waves.

more

6. With atrial rates much over 400 per minute, the atria simply _____ because they can't respond to so many stimuli.

twitch

7. This is called _____ _____.

atrial fibrillation

8. In this case, impulses reach the AV node irregularly, so conduction to the ventricles is _____ too.

irregular

9. As a result, the ventricular rhythm becomes _____.

irregular

10. Thus, in atrial arrhythmias the ventricular rate and rhythm are determined by the number of _____ impulses and whether they are blocked at the _____ _____.

atrial   AV node

Review 3

Although *The Manual* stresses the danger of atrial arrhythmias, it is important to realize that some people live all their lives with these conditions. So let's discuss the etiology of atrial arrhythmias and find out just when they are dangerous.

1. Irritability of atrial cells is usually due to _____ or _____ _____.

ischemia   atrial overdistention

2. This irritability leads to atrial _____.

arrhythmias

3. Atrial arrhythmias can cause the ventricular rate to _____ greatly.

increase

4. Very rapid ventricular rates can cause a _____ in cardiac output.

decrease

5. Why? _____

Because the time for ventricular filling is shortened.

6. These atrial arrhythmias would be considered _____ arrhythmias if they occurred after an MI.

dangerous or major

7. If a patient has been in normal sinus rhythm before an MI and develops atrial arrhythmias after an MI, these (should/should not) be treated.

should

8. Why? _____

Because they may reduce cardiac output.

9. If a patient has lived with atrial fibrillation for years before an MI, the atrial arrhythmia probably (does/does not) have to be treated (except to control rapid ventricular rates).

does not

10. The great danger of atrial arrhythmias is the fast _____ rate they may produce.

ventricular

11. The atrial contraction contributes about _____% to cardiac output.

20

12. So when the atria fibrillate (eg, twitch) and don't pump, it is described as "losing the atrial _____."

kick

PREMATURE ATRIAL CONTRACTIONS (pp. 156–159)

I would like to introduce you to the triplets, PAC, PJC, and PVC. PAC is probably the least troublesome of the three. You will meet the other two later.

Review 4

1. A premature baby comes _____ he is expected.   before

2. Premature beats come _____ the normal beat is expected.   before

3. A premature beat is an (ectopic/normal) beat.   ectopic

4. Ectopic beats can come from _____ areas (foci) in the heart.   irritable

5. PACs come from irritable foci in the _____.   atria

6. The patient usually (does/does not) feel these beats.   does not

7. PACs are diagnosed by _____.   ECG

8. You (would/would not) see a P wave with a PAC.   would

9. The configuration of the P wave with a PAC (would/would not) be normal.   would not

10. PACs (are/are not) inherently dangerous.   are not

11. PACs may warn of increasing atrial _____.   irritability

12. Suppose you have had a normal beat and almost immediately an irritable ectopic atrial focus fires. The AV node may not be _____ and ready to conduct (ie, it may still be refractory).   repolarized

13. Would you see a normal PQRST?   no

14. Now fire that ectopic impulse after the AV node is repolarized but while portions of the His bundle–Purkinji system are still refractory. You would expect (slower/faster) than normal conduction and a QRS of (less than/more than) .12 seconds.   slower / more than

15. With your stethoscope you may hear a louder than usual _____ heart sound because the premature contraction catches the _____-_____ valve leaflets further apart than usual at systole.   first / atrio-ventricular

16. Positive identification of this arrhythmia can only be made by _____.   ECG

PAROXYSMAL SUPRAVENTRICULAR TACHYCARDIA (pp. 160–163)

"In the beginning" we had simple PAT, caused by an irritable atrial focus. Then they did more studies and lo and behold! we were only right 10% of the time. Now it's believed that 90% of PSVT is caused by re-entry loops. (Stay tuned—the 6th edition will probably bring more changes!) Anyway, let's plunge in and re-orient our thinking to re-entry. Let's start with what we know.

Review 5

1. A tachycardia is a continuous heart rate over _____ per minute.   100

2. The T in PSVT stands for _____.   tachycardia

3. Paroxysmal means to start and stop _____.   suddenly

4. Sinus tachycardia is usually paroxysmal. (True/False)   False

5. SV tachycardia is usually paroxysmal. (True/False)   True

6. The atrial rate in PAT (the 10%) is usually _____ to _____ per minute.   150 250

7. The ventricular rate in PAT is usually _____ to _____ per minute.   150 250

8. PAT is caused by an irritable _____ _____. | atrial focus

9. You know that supraventricular (SV) means _____ the ventricles. | above

10. 90% of PSVT is due to _____ loops. | re-entry

11. Four possible sites for re-entry loops are:

    a. _____ | SA node

    b. _____ | atria

    c. _____ | AV node

    d. _____ | accessory bypass tracts

12. An accessory bypass tract is one that connects the atria directly to the ventricles, by-passing the _____ node. | AV

13. In order for a re-entry loop to occur, there must be (1/2/3/4) functionally different tracts. | 2

14. Let's take them one at a time. One tract must conduct _____ and have a short refractory period. | slowly

15. The other conducts more rapidly and has a _____ refractory period. | longer

16. An impulse may conduct down one pathway, find the other pathway repolarized and be conducted _____ initiating a _____ loop. | retrograde   re-entry

17. The ventricles respond to _____ atrial impulse so atrial and ventricular rates are the _____ (unless an AV block exists). | each / same

18. Patients usually (can/cannot) feel PSVT. | can

19. A rapid PSVT can (increase/decrease) cardiac output. | decrease

20. Decreased cardiac output can cause _____ _____ _____. | left ventricular failure

21. Rapid ventricular rates can (increase/decrease) myocardial oxygen demand. | increase

22. Increased demand and decreased output can cause myocardial _____. | ischemia

23. Myocardial ischemia can cause _____. | angina

24. After an MI, PSVT (is/is not) dangerous. | is

25. The longer PSVT lasts, the _____ the danger. | greater

26. PSVT can sometimes be stopped by pressure on the _____ _____ or the _____ (reflex vagal stimulation). | carotid sinuses / eyeballs

27. Vagal stimulation (increases/decreases) parasympathetic effect (ie, more slowing down) on the AV node. This (increases/decreases) AV conduction and breaks the re-entry circuit. | increases / decreases

28. If PSVT does not cause distress, drugs (especially IV _____) may be tried. | adenosine

29. This drug slows conduction through the _____ and _____ nodes and can interrupt the _____ pathways. | SA   AV / re-entry

30. Other drugs used include calcium-blocking agents (eg, _____) and beta-blocking agents (eg, _____). | verapamil / propranolol

31. These drugs also (slow/speed up) conduction through the _____ and _____ nodes and block _____ circuits. | slow   SA / AV   re-entry

32. Rapid-acting _____ can be used but it has a slower onset of action. | digitalis

33. If PSVT causes angina or symptoms, elective _____ _____ should be used immediately. | precordial shock

34. For the 10% of true PAT, _____ toxicity and (hypokalemia/hyperkalemia) should be suspected. | digitalis   hypokalemia

ATRIAL FLUTTER *(pp. 164–166)*

Review 6

1. In atrial flutter, the pacemaker is an ectopic focus in the _____.

   atria

2. The rate of this atrial focus is _____ to _____ per minute.

   250   400

3. The AV node protects the ventricle from this rapid rate by _____ some of the atrial impulses.

   blocking

4. True P waves are replaced by _____ waves.

   flutter

5. There are (more/fewer) flutter waves than QRSs.

   more

6. Generally you can count out a ratio of _____ waves to _____ waves.

   atrial or flutter
   ventricular

7. There may be a 2:1, 3:1, 4:1 atrial/ventricular _____.

   block

8. The patient's block (can/cannot) change.

   can

9. If it changes, the ventricular rate will be (regular/irregular).

   irregular

10. You already know that rapid ventricular rates decrease _____ _____, and cause myocardial _____ and _____.

    cardiac output
    ischemia   angina

11. An unusual risk is if the atrial rate slows to where the AV node, instead of blocking, can conduct _____ impulse, leaving a rapid, ineffective _____ rate.

    each   ventricular

12. _____-channel-blocking agents may convert the rhythm or reduce the flutter rate.

    Sodium

13. Then other drugs must be given to (increase/decrease) the AV block and prevent too rapid a ventricular rate.

    increase

14. Some of these drugs are digitalis, _____-blockers and _____-channel-blockers.

    beta   calcium

15. A temporary _____ may be used to break the re-entry circuit.

    pacemaker

16. Atrial flutter is a dangerous arrhythmia if the ventricular rate is _____.

    rapid

17. The surest treatment for atrial flutter is _____ _____.

    synchronized shock

18. Thought question: Your patient is in atrial flutter with a ventricular rate of about 80. He is in no discomfort. Why would you monitor him closely? _____ _____ _____

    Atrial flutter blocks are variable; his ventricular rate can change at any time if the AV block changes.

ATRIAL FIBRILLATION *(pp. 167–171)*

Review 7

1. Atrial fibrillation is caused by ectopic foci and multiple re-entry loops in the _____.

   atria

2. The atrial rate of over _____ per minute causes the atria to merely twitch.

   400

3. The AV node is bombarded by these atrial impulses: it conducts (regularly/irregularly) to the ventricles.

   irregularly

4. If the ventricular response is over 100 per minute, it is called _____ atrial fibrillation.

   rapid

5. If the ventricular rate is below 100 per minute, it is called _____ atrial fibrillation.

   slow

6. Rapid ventricular rates _____ the threat of left ventricular failure.

   increase

7. The apical (heart) rate is usually (more/less) than the radial (pulse) rate.

8. Thus, if an unmonitored patient has a totally irregular pulse, you should take the _____ rate.

9. The difference between apical and radial pulse is called _____ _____.

10. Finding a pulse deficit on an unmonitored patient with an irregular pulse might make you suspect he has _____ _____.

11. The atria (do/do not) contract in atrial fibrillation.

12. The loss of atrial contraction _____ ventricular output by about 20%.

13. Decreased ventricular filling may also contribute to left ventricular _____, and myocardial _____.

14. Blood clots tend to form in the noncontracting _____.

15. Uncontrolled atrial fibrillation (is/is not) a dangerous arrhythmia when it occurs after an MI.

16. Atrial fibrillation that is causing complications should be terminated with _____ _____.

17. If atrial fibrillation is treated with drugs, the first objective is to _____ the ventricular rate by _____ the AV block.

18. Drugs used for this are _____, _____-_____, and _____ channel blockers.

19. Then an _____ drug must be given to break the _____ circuit and convert the rhythm to normal.

20. Esmolol is a rapid-acting _____-_____ given as a 0.5 mg/kg _____, followed by a 0.05 mg/kg _____ for rapid control of atrial fibrillation. (Consult your drug book on Esmolol, it's interesting reading.)

On the ECG there are two hallmarks of atrial fibrillation: an irregular, indefinable baseline (a "messy" baseline), and total irregularity of the R waves. Remember these two, and please note: the ventricular rate and/or width of the QRS is not part of the criteria for diagnosis of atrial fibrillation.

I would like to give you a hint on how to check an ECG for regularity of the heartbeat. Sometimes you can't be sure by simply looking at the R waves, and you need a more exact method. One way of doing this is to use measuring calipers, which should be part of the equipment in a CCU. But since you might not carry these with you, all you have to do is lay a piece of scrap paper across the rhythm strip so that the R waves show above it. Now make marks on the scrap paper where the first three R waves appear. Then slide the paper to the right so that the mark on the first R wave is now on the third R wave. If the rhythm is regular, the marks will fall directly on succeeding R waves. If they don't, you know the rhythm is irregular.

Try this method on the following ECG. Is the rhythm regular or irregular?

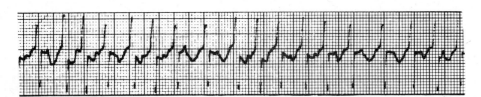

Figure 10.1

ATRIAL STANDSTILL *(pp. 172–174)*

Review 8

Look at the rhythm strip on page 173 in *The Manual*. Can you find any P waves? (I hope not!) As you know, the P waves show depolarization of the atria, and obviously these atria are just sitting—or standing—there.

1. The normal pacemaker is the _____ _____.

   SA node

2. If it fails, we hope the _____ will generate impulses.

   atria

3. Sudden loss of P waves on the monitor can be a warning of impending atrial _____.

   standstill

4. With loss of atrial activity, the pacemaker descends to the _____ _____ or (junctional) area.

   AV nodal

5. Failure of the junctional area leaves only the _____ pacemakers to initiate impulses.

   ventricular

6. This progression is called _____ displacement of the pacemaker.

   downward

7. Downward displacement may be associated with left _____ _____ or cardiogenic _____.

   ventricular failure shock

8. Overdosages of _____ and _____ can cause downward displacement of the pacemaker.

   digitalis quinidine

9. Electrolyte imbalances, _____, can also cause atrial standstill.

   hyperkalemia

10. However, the usual cause is irreversible damage to higher _____ centers.

    pacemaker

11. Atrial standstill is an ominous warning of progressive _____ _____ of the pacemaker.

    downward displacement

12. Lower pacemaker centers are inherently (slower/faster) and (less/just as) reliable than higher centers.

    slower less

13. Primary treatment is to institute _____ _____.

    transvenous pacing

MONITOR PRACTICE

Review 9

It seems to me that atrial arrhythmias are more interesting than any of the others. They are less lethal than ventricular arrhythmias, and some of them look downright pretty on the monitor. All of the following example strips are from patients who had MIs. Fill in the answers.

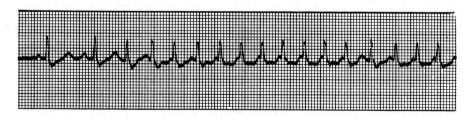

Figure 10.2. Mr. Whoops.

It's breakfast time in CCU. Things are quiet, when suddenly the high-rate alarm rings.

1. The first two beats originate in the _____ _____.

   SA node

2. Then, whoops! He develops _____ _____ _____.

   paroxysmal supraventricular tachycardia

3. The rapid rate may cause _____.

4. If sustained, it may lead to _____ _____ _____.

5. Would you observe this arrhythmia for a few minutes, or call the doctor stat? Why?
_____
_____
_____
_____
_____

6. This is a lethal arrhythmia. (True/False)

7. If this arrhythmia recurs, you would anticipate using which of the following: atropine, rapid-acting digitalis, Isuprel, adenosine, verapamil, nitroglycerin, or propranolol.
_____

Review 10

He was just admitted, and has no symptoms now. You take an admission rhythm strip and see the following ECG. Insignificant looking, isn't it? Better look carefully.

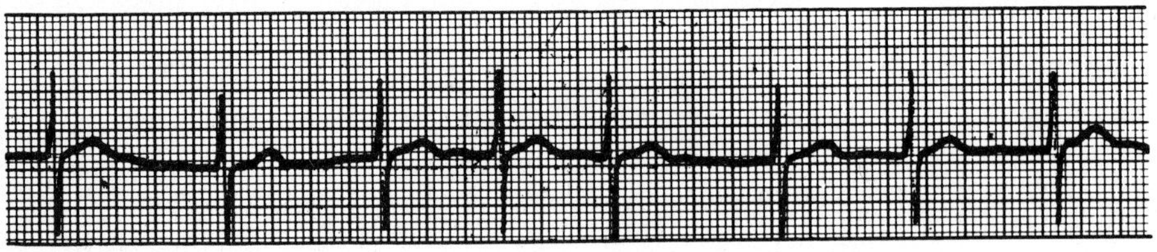

Figure 10.3. Mr. Ho-Hum.

1. Are P waves present and normal? _____.

2. What does that tell you? _____
_____.

3. Are the R–R times regular? _____.

4. No P waves and totally irregular R–R = _____.

5. What is the ventricular rate? _____

6. Is this rapid atrial fibrillation? _____
_____
_____.

7. Should you document the arrhythmia? _____

8. Should you call the doctor stat? _____
_____
_____.

9. You would want to ask the patient if he has been taking _____.

10. What is the most important factor in deciding whether the arrhythmia should be treated? _____
_____.

11. Could this arrhythmia have been present for many years and not be related to myocardial infarction? _____
_____.

angina

left ventricular failure

Observe for a few minutes. It may stop spontaneously. Besides, you want to see if the patient develops any symptoms with the tachycardia.

False

rapid-acting digitalis, adenosin, verapamil, propranolol

No P waves are present

The pacemaker is *not* in the SA node

No, they are irregular

atrial fibrillation

80 per minute

No, it's slow, since ventricular rate is less than 100 per minute

Yes

No, this isn't an emergency. Call the doctor after you have all the admission information

digitalis

Whether or not the patient has left ventricular failure

Yes, some patients have atrial fibrillation. And it may have no connection with the acute MI

Review 11

The QRS complexes are inverted because of the position of the chest electrodes.

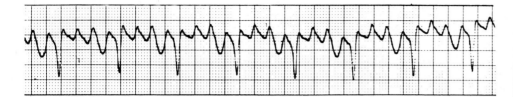

Figure 10.4. Ms. Rick-Rack.

1. ECG interpretation: _____ _____.

   atrial flutter

2. The atrial focus is discharging at a rate of _____ per minute (or _____ flutter waves in _____ seconds).

   320   32
   6

3. The ventricular rate is _____.

   80 per minute

4. This means the _____ node is blocking some atrial impulses to protect the ventricle.

   AV

5. What is the ratio of flutter waves (F waves) to R waves? _____

   4:1

6. Are the R–R times regular? _____

   Yes

7. Would they be in atrial fibrillation? _____.

   No, they would be irregular in atrial fibrillation

8. Drug therapy must _____ the atrial rate without allowing the ventricular rate to _____.

   slow
   increase

9. The ventricular rate can be controlled by increasing the degree of _____ block.

   AV

Review 12

He has been in the CCU for two days. He has had signs of mild left ventricular failure, but no digitalis has been given. Today he developed this arrhythmia.

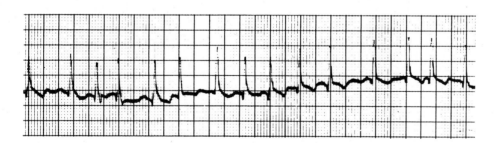

Figure 10.5. Mr. A.F.

1. What is the ventricular rate? _____.

   150 per minute

2. Is the rhythm regular? _____.

   No, it's irregular

3. Is the baseline regular? _____.

   No, the baseline varies

4. ECG diagnosis: _____ _____.

   atrial fibrillation

5. Is the ventricular rate "slow"? _____.

   No, it's rapid

6. This arrhythmia may _____ the pumping efficiency of the heart.

   decrease

7. Since the patient already has left ventricular failure, it may get _____.

worse

8. With this patient in distress, the best treatment is _____ _____ _____ _____.

synchronized precordial shock (cardioversion)

Now that you have interpreted the rhythm strips, draw a big breath. You have completed sinus and atrial arrhythmias and should be quite proud of yourself.

11

Arrhythmias Originating
in the AV Junction

Review 1

1. In "downward displacement" of the pacemaker, the pacemaker may "escape" from the SA node to the _____ _____ area.

   AV   junctional

2. The area where the AV node joins the bundle of His is called the _____ area.

   junctional

3. The junctional area (can/cannot) initiate impulses.

   can

4. Thus, arrhythmias originating in the AV nodal/bundle of His area are called _____ arrhythmias.

   junctional

5. The junctional area's inherent discharge rate is (slower/faster) than the SA node.

   slower

6. If the junctional area takes over as pacemaker, you would expect a rate of about _____ to _____ per minute.

   40   60

7. This would be called a _____ rhythm or a junctional _____ rhythm.

   junctional   escape

8. Junctional rhythm occurs when _____ pacing centers are depressed.

   higher

9. Increased activity of the junctional area can lead to faster _____ rhythms (above 60/min.).

   junctional

10. In general, rapid rates are called _____.

    tachycardias

11. A tachycardia that starts and stops suddenly is called a _____ tachycardia.

    paroxysmal

12. A fast-rate arrhythmia originating paroxysmally in the junctional tissue would be called _____ junctional tachycardia.

    paroxysmal

13. If the tachycardia began gradually, it could be termed non-_____ junctional tachycardia (NPJT).

    paroxysmal

14. Another name for NPJT is _____ _____ _____.

    accelerated junctional rhythm

15. Ectopic premature beats originating from around the junctional area are called _____ _____ _____ abbreviated as _____.

    premature junctional contractions   PJC

147

16. If the SA node and atria fail to discharge impulses, downward displacement of the pacemaker occurs and the _____ _____ is next in line to serve as pacemaker.

junctional area

17. This could happen after _____ to the higher centers.

injury or ischemia

18. Thus, junctional arrhythmias (except PJCs) are considered (major/minor) arrhythmias.

major

PREMATURE JUNCTIONAL CONTRACTIONS (pp. 180–182)

Review 2

How about some What, Where, Why, When questions? Let's start off with the cause of PJC.

1. An ectopic focus in the _____ area can initiate an impulse _____ the
   _{where}   _{when}
   SA impulse.

junctional   before

2. This stimulus is transmitted _____ through the _____ system
   _{where}   _{what}
   and produces ventricular _____.
   _{what}

downward   His–Purkinje
depolarization

3. The ectopic junctional impulse can also go _____ and _____ the atria.
   _{where}   _{what}

upward   depolarize

4. If atrial depolarization precedes ventricular depolarization, you will see a _____
   _{what}
   before the QRS on the ECG.

P wave

5. If atrial and ventricular depolarization are simultaneous, the _____ can be
   _{what}
   "buried" in the _____ and not be visible.
   _{where}

P wave
QRS

6. If the atria depolarize *after* the ventricles, on the ECG you will see a _____ wave
   _{what}
   first and then a _____.
   _{what}

QRS
P wave

7. Since atrial depolarization is from the "bottom up" or retrograde, the P waves may appear _____ (or "upside down").
   _{how}

inverted

8. PJCs are caused by _____ of the junctional tissue, probably due to
   _{what}
   _____.
   _{what}

irritability
ischemia

9. PJCs (are/are not) considered serious or major arrhythmias.

are not

Review 3

Ms. Pre Junque is a 95-pound, 85-year-old antique dealer, a post-MI in your unit. You begin noticing premature ectopic beats on the monitor. What would you do?

1. _____ the arrhythmia by running a rhythm strip.

Document

2. _____ the patient's clinical status by inquiring how she feels. ("Just fine, Honey, just fine.")

Assess

3. _____ her vital signs ("Y'all gonna wear my poor ole arm out, Honey").

Check

4. Study the monitor strip, looking especially at the relationship of _____ waves and _____ complexes.

P
QRS

5. It is important to differentiate PJCs from _____.

PVCs

6. If you aren't sure whether it is a PVC or PJC, you may need to get a _____ _____.

12-lead ECG

7. While Ms. Junque raves about the market for antique shoehorns, you continue to evaluate the situation. The ectopics are increasing. You get ready to administer either _____ IV or _____ and call the doctor.

lidocaine   procainamide

148

JUNCTIONAL RHYTHM (pp. 183–185)

Review 4

When the higher pacemakers are depressed, the junctional area can take over at rates below 60 per minute and pace the heart. Is this a problem? Does it make any difference who pitches, as long as we have a ball game? Suppose we think this through.

1. In junctional rhythm the pacemaker is in the _____ _____.

junctional tissue

2. It paces at a rate of about _____ to _____ beats per minute.

40 60

3. Junctional rhythm is possible when the SA node is _____.

depressed

4. The SA node may be depressed due to increased _____ stimulation.

vagal

5. Other causes of SA depression may be _____ or overdoses of _____ or _____.

ischemia digitalis
quinidine

6. Junctional rhythm can only be diagnosed for certain by _____.

ECG

7. Junctional rhythm is often (temporary/permanent).

temporary

8. However, any slow rhythm is dangerous because of _____ cardiac output.

decreased

9. Junctional pacemakers are _____ dependable.

not

10. Another danger is that faster, irritable ectopic foci may _____ _____ as pacemaker.

take over

11. Junctional rhythm may be a _____ of more serious arrhythmias.

warning or forerunner

12. There (is/is no) specific drug therapy for slow junctional rhythm; _____ may be tried to stimulate SA nodal discharge.

is no atropine

13. Transvenous _____ may be used to increase the rate and the cardiac output.

pacing

14. Lidocaine usually (is/is not) effective in suppressing ectopic beats occurring with slow junctional rhythm.

is not

PAROXYSMAL JUNCTIONAL TACHYCARDIA (pp. 186–189)

Review 5

1. Paroxysmal junctional tachycardia (PJT, please) is the (most/least) common form of PSVT.

most

2. Paroxysmal tachycardias whether originating in the atria or junctional area, _____ and _____ suddenly.

begin
stop

3. PSVT (atrial or junctional) have a regular, rapid rate of _____ to _____ per minute.

140 250

4. 90% of the time the cause is a _____ _____ in the AV _____.

re-entry loop node

5. In PSVT impulses conduct normally through the ventricles (so you would see a normal _____ on the monitor), but conduction is _____ back through the atria. So you may see P waves that occur _____, _____, or _____ the QRS.

QRS retrograde
before during after

6. Thought question: How can you tell there is a P wave buried in a QRS? You can't see it. _____ _____.

   Answer: Mark out P waves with calipers or scrap paper. If Ps occur regularly but one is missing where a QRS is, you assume the missing P wave is just hiding, obscured by the QRS.

149

7. The most probable cause of PJT is _____ of the AV node.

ischemia

8. Other secondary causes of PJT include _____ toxicity, _____ disturbances, and increased _____ secretion.

digitalis metabolic
catecholamine

Review 6

Let's take a good look at the mechanism of re-entry; if you gloss over it now, I guarantee, it will drive you crazy later on.

1. Be sure you understand that the re-entry pathways we are discussing are NOT in the _____ branches, NOT in the two fascicles of the _____ bundle branch, NOT even in the bundle of _____.

bundle left
His

2. They are in the _____ node itself.

AV

3. Call them pathways A and B. Most of the time impulses go down (A/B/both).

both

4. Say that conduction down B is faster, so that this impulse _____ the bundle of His. "Good Ole His" now needs a rest; ie, "His" is _____ to further stimulation until he _____.

depolarizes
refractory
repolarizes

5. So now an impulse coming down A (where it conducts more _____), finds the bundle of His _____ and the impulse is simply blocked.

slowly
refractory

6. To summarize: B conducts _____ but has a _____ refractory period.

faster longer

7. Pathway A conducts _____ but its refractory period is _____.

slower shorter

8. Suppose the normal SA impulse has gone down B and B is now refractory. Fire off a PAC. Pathway A with its shorter _____ period may (accept/block) the PAC.

refractory accept

9. Now A conducts (slower/faster) so by the time the PAC stimulus reaches the bundle of His, B may be _____ and accept the PAC's stimulus.

slower
repolarized

10. The impulse can then go _____ back up B and find (slow/fast) repolarizing A ready to accept the stimulus again.

retrogradely fast

11. This can create a sustained _____ rhythm.

re-entry

12. The big problem is that the _____ are also stimulated by each junctional impulse.

ventricles

13. Any rapid ventricular rhythm is dangerous because it causes (increased/decreased) cardiac output, (increased/decreased) myocardial oxygen demand, and decreased coronary artery filling because there is (less/more) time to fill during (diastole/systole).

decreased
increased
less diastole

14. All of number 13 can cause further _____ damage and ultimately _____ ventricular failure.

ischemic
left

15. The patient often experiences _____, _____, and _____.

angina dyspnea
apprehension

16. A tachycardia of 140 to 250/min. with questionable P waves means you need a _____ for diagnosis.

12-lead ECG

17. It is often impossible to differentiate PJT from other PSVT, but the treatment is the same: _____ _____ _____ is tried first.

carotid sinus massage

18. If the patient is not in distress, you might give IV _____.

adenosine

19. However, this drug is not used in tachycardias caused by _____ ectopic foci because its main action is slowing conduction through the _____ and _____ nodes.

ventricular
SA
AV

20. How can you be certain what kind of tachycardia you are seeing? _____

12-lead ECG

21. Other drugs that might be tried are _____ channel blockers (eg, _____), beta-blockers (eg, _____).

calcium verapamil
propranolol

22. Carotid sinus massage and the drugs mentioned all work by (slowing/speeding up) AV conduction and blocking _____ _____.

> slowing
> re-entry circuits

23. Sustained PJT with definite symptoms must be terminated immediately with _____ _____ _____, also known as _____.

> synchronized precordial shock
> cardioversion

24. If a patient has a short burst of PJT that subsides spontaneously, should he have antiarrhythmic therapy? _____

> Yes

25. Drugs used include _____, _____, _____, and _____ _____.

> propranolol   quinidine
> digitalis   calcium blockers

NONPAROXYSMAL JUNCTIONAL TACHYCARDIA (pp. 190–192)

Review 7

1. The inherent pacing rate of junctional tissue is _____ to _____ beats per minute.

> 40   60

2. If the junctional area initiates impulses faster than 60 beats per minute, you could term it a _____ for the junctional cells.

> tachycardia

3. The rates in non-paroxysmal tachycardia are between _____ and _____ beats per minute.

> 70   130

4. A more appropriate name might be _____ _____ rhythm.

> accelerated junctional

5. NPJT often is associated with _____ _____ _____ and _____ _____.

> advanced heart failure
> cardiogenic shock

6. It can also be caused by _____.

> digitalis

7. If you continued to give digitalis to a patient with NPJT what might happen? _____ _____ _____

> atrial fibrillation, heart block, ventricular standstill

8. Other possible causes of NPJT are acute _____ MI, _____ (from rheumatic fever), cardiac _____, and congenital anomalies.

> inferior   myocarditis
> surgery

9. NPJT often warns of further _____ displacement of the pacemaker.

> downward

10. Symptoms are usually related to _____ _____ _____ _____ _____.

> left ventricular failure
>   (or CHF)

11. There (is/is not) a specific treatment for NPJT.

> is not

12. _____ _____ may be used because of the danger of downward displacement of the pacemaker.

> Transvenous pacing

13. An attempt may be made to slow the ventricular rate by giving _____, _____, or _____.

> quinidine
>   procainamide   propranolol

PUTTING IT TOGETHER

Review 8

Okay, back to your make-believe CCU. You have identified a change in a patient's monitor pattern. The P waves are inverted and the P–R intervals are short. The QRS is normal.

1. To begin with, you should decide if the monitor is showing a _____ rhythm.

> junctional

2. Now consider the rate. If the rate is between 40 and 60, you probably are seeing _____ _____.

> junctional rhythm

3. If the rate is between 70 and 130, the patient is likely to have _____.

> NPJT

4. A rate of 140 to 220 would indicate a _____.

5. If the QRS is normal and the rate isn't too bad, you do not need to bother the doctor at night about this. (True/False)

6. Junctional rhythm and tachycardias (are/are not) considered warnings of impending danger.

7. If the patient's dose of digitalis is due, you would want to _____
_____.

8. If the junctional rhythm is slow, you could anticipate that the doctor might want to
_____.

False. You'd better!

are

consult the doctor before giving it

insert a transvenous pacemaker

12

Arrhythmias Originating in the Ventricles

When the pacemaker of an ischemic heart has retreated to the ventricles, there is not much room for further downward displacement. This is it; the bottom of the totem pole. And while infrequent, single focus (unifocal) PVCs may not be dangerous, they certainly keep nurses alert! Let's learn when to chew our fingernails and when to defibrillate.

VENTRICULAR ARRHYTHMIAS

Review 1

1. An arrhythmia originating above the ventricles is called _____.

    supraventricular

2. Ventricular arrhythmias start below the _____ _____ _____.

    AV nodal area

3. Normal people may have PVCs that cause no problem. (True/False)

    True

4. PVCs are dangerous for the patient who has had an _____.

    AMI

5. The progression of dangerous arrhythmias is: premature _____ contractions → ventricular _____ → ventricular _____.

    ventricular
    tachycardia   fibrillation

6. The rate of ventricular tachycardia is _____ to _____ per minute.

    140   250

7. Ventricular tachycardia is really a series of _____ (3 or more).

    PVCs

8. If you see on the monitor a rhythm that looks like ventricular tachycardia with a rate of 50 to 100/minute, you would call it _____ _____ rhythm.

    accelerated
    idioventricular

9. This ventricular arrhythmia (does/does not) lead to ventricular fibrillation.

    does not

10. Ventricular tachycardia (does/does not) lead to ventricular fibrillation.

    does

11. So if you see what appears to be a continual string of PVCs you should _____ _____ _____.

    count the rate

12. "Ratewise" (under/over) 100 is not so dangerous; (under/over) 140 is dangerous.

    under   over

PREMATURE VENTRICULAR CONTRACTIONS *(pp. 198–200)*

For a long time I have been promising that we would learn more about PVCs and ventricular fibrillation. The time has come.

Review 2

1. A contraction occurring before the regularly expected sinus beat is _____.

   premature

2. A PVC is a premature contraction originating from an irritable focus in the _____.

   ventricle

3. The most common ventricular arrhythmia is the _____.

   PVC

4. The most common of *all* arrhythmias is the _____ (ie, in AMI patients).

   PVC

5. In PVCs the QRS will be (wide/narrow).

   wide

6. A wide QRS measures more than _____ second.

   0.12

7. The QRS will be (normal/abnormal) in shape.

   abnormal

8. The abnormal QRS is described as _____ in shape.

   distorted

9. The T wave usually (is/is not) the opposite direction from the QRS of the PVC.

   is

10. Thus, if the PVC had a negative (downward) QRS, the T wave probably would be _____.

    positive (upright)

11. If the PVC has a positive (upright) QRS, the T wave probably would be _____ (*Note:* Questions 10 and 11 are "probably," not absolutely.)

    negative (downward)

12. Measuring from the normal QRS before the PVC to the normal QRS after the PVC should equal _____ R–R intervals.

    two

13. This delay after a PVC is called a full _____ _____.

    compensatory pause

14. In summary: PVCs can be diagnosed by a QRS that is _____ in shape and over _____ wide.

    distorted
    0.12 seconds

15. The T wave is probably in the _____ direction from the QRS, and there should be a full _____ _____.

    opposite
    compensatory pause

16. The QRS is widened and distorted because conduction through the ventricles is _____ _____ _____ and not through the normal _____ system.

    cell to cell   conduction

Treatment of PVCs *(p. 200)*
Review 3

1. The primary drug treatment for PVCs is _____.

   lidocaine

2. A trade name for lidocaine is _____.

   Xylocaine

3. Initially, lidocaine is given as a _____ dose, IV.

   push or bolus

4. The usual push dosage is _____ to _____ mg.

   50   100

5. Lidocaine should then be continued as an IV _____, 2 to 3 mg/min.

   drip

6. An overdose of lidocaine can cause _____.

   convulsions

7. If lidocaine fails, _____ can be tried.

   procainamide

8. Procainamide and Pronestyl (are/are not) the same.

   are

9. Pronestyl may cause the blood pressure to (drop/rise).

   drop

10. Antiarrhythmic drugs sometimes (rarely) used to control PVCs are _____, _____, and _____. | quinidine disopyramide   flecainide

11. Oral agents (should/should not) be used for emergency treatment of PVCs. | should not

12. Potassium (can/cannot) be used to suppress PVCs. One rule of thumb about treating PVCs: total lidocaine should not exceed 500 mg/hour. Respect lidocaine: the convulsions brought on by an overdose are unbelievable. Respect Pronestyl: your patient's blood pressure can "fall through the floor" with it. | can

FIVE DANGEROUS FORMS OF PREMATURE VENTRICULAR CONTRACTIONS *(pp. 201–203)*

Now that we can recognize PVCs, we need to know when to intelligently fear them. The figures in *The Manual,* Chapter 12, are beautiful guides for recognizing different types of PVCs. Study these pages carefully. If you can't diagnose PVCs, you will be miserable as a CCU nurse.

Review 4

1. PVCs usually indicate ventricular _____. | irritability

2. They may also be caused by drugs, especially _____. | digitalis

3. Patients with a low level of the electrolyte _____ tend to develop PVCs. | potassium

4. Potassium may be depleted during _____ therapy. | diuretic

5. Low potassium is called _____. | hypokalemia

6. Isolated, infrequent PVCs usually (are/are not) dangerous. | are not

7. Increasing numbers of PVCs indicate (increasing/decreasing) irritability. | increasing

8. Increased ventricular irritability can lead to ventricular _____. | tachycardia

9. Ventricular tachycardia can progress to ventricular _____. | fibrillation

10. You know how many PVCs per minute your patient has because you _____ them on the monitor. Which is more dangerous, two PVCs per minute or seven per minute? _____ | count (document) seven

11. If you see _____ or more PVCs a minute, you would consider them very dangerous. | six

12. If every other beat is a PVC, the rhythm is called _____. | bigeminy

13. Ventricular bigeminy (is/is not) dangerous. | is

14. A PVC falling on the _____-wave of the preceding QRS is particularly dangerous. | T

15. This is called an _____-_____-_____ pattern. | R-on-T

16. PVCs originating from more than one ectopic focus are called _____. | multifocal

17. How do you know they come from more than one focus? _____ | Because of the differences in the configuration of the PVC.

18. Multifocal PVCs are usually (more/less) dangerous than unifocal PVCs. | more

19. _____ consecutive PVCs, known as couplets or _____, are especially dangerous. | Two   pairs

20. In summary, the dangerous PVCs are:

    A. _____ or more per minute. | six

    B. _____ (every other beat) | bigeminal

C. _____-_____-_____ pattern,   R-on-T

D. _____-focal, and   multi

E. _____ or more in a row.   two

21. There is a higher mortality in AMI patients who have more than _____ PVCs per   10
minute, _____, or _____.   couplets   triplets

VENTRICULAR TACHYCARDIA *(pp. 204–208)*

PVCs → ventricular tachycardia → ventricular fibrillation: a progression you will do
your best to stop. Though ventricular tachycardia is in the middle of the scale, it's defi-
nitely an acute emergency (and that's worse than a plain emergency)! The ECGs in *The
Manual,* Chapter 12, depict ventricular tachycardia beautifully. Study them and don't forget them!

Review 5

1. Ventricular tachycardia is defined as _____ or more PVCs in a row (at a rate of   three
140 to 250/min).

2. It is caused by severe _____ irritability.   ventricular

3. Ventricular tachycardia is often an immediate forerunner of _____   ventricular
_____.   fibrillation

4. Ventricular tachycardia (may/may not) occur in short runs or bursts.   may

5. This is called nonsustained VT.   True

6. Persistent, sustained VT is less of a threat.   False

7. With sustained ventricular tachycardia, cardiac output is likely to _____.   fall

8. Decreased cardiac output may lead to _____ _____ failure.   left ventricular

9. Or worse, it may lead to _____ _____.   cardiogenic shock

10. Ventricular tachycardia can suddenly change to _____ _____.   ventricular fibrillation

11. All of this means that ventricular tachycardia is an extremely _____ ar-   dangerous
rhythmia.

Review 6

1. If ventricular tachycardia stops abruptly, you can sit back and forget about it.
(True/False)   False

2. There is a (low/high) risk of further episodes.   high

3. Why? _____ .   The underlying problem is still
                                                             present

4. Therefore treatment is necessary to prevent _____ _____.   further attacks

5. Ventricular tachycardia is treated with _____.   lidocaine

6. The initial treatment is a push dose containing _____ mg.   100

7. After the push dose, continue lidocaine in an _____ _____. (3000 mg in 500 cc   IV drip
at 2 to 4 mg/min).

8. Some doctors use _____ _____ if lidocaine fails (adrenergic an-   bretylium tosylate
tagonist, sympatholytic).

9. If ventricular tachycardia continues despite the push dose of lidocaine, the next step
is _____ _____.   precordial shock

10. Repeated attacks of this arrhythmia may be due to an electrolyte imbalance called _____.

11. This means low _____.

12. It would be wise to have the _____ at the bedside once a patient has had ventricular tachycardia.

13. _____ _____ could develop very suddenly.

hypokalemia

potassium

defibrillator

Ventricular fibrillation

MONITOR PRACTICE (PVCs AND VENTRICULAR TACHYCARDIA)

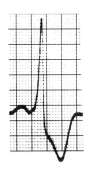

Figure 12.1

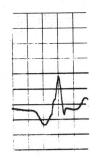

Figure 12.2

Review 7

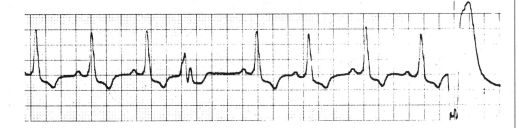

Figure 12.3. Mr. P.B.

1. In six seconds our patient has had _____ PVCs.

2. Assuming he continues at this rate, he will have _____ PVCs per minute.

3. You treat PVCs when they are over _____ per minute so give him a bolus of _____—fast!

4. How many foci of PVCs do you see? _____

5. Multifocal PVCs are _____ dangerous than unifocal. It shouldn't surprise you too much that this irritable heart went into ventricular tachycardia in the middle of the night. (He responded to lidocaine, recovered, and eventually went home.)

two

20

six
lidocaine

Two

more

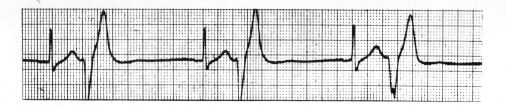

Figure 12.4. Mr. B. Jimminy.

6. Every other beat is a _____ _____ _____.

premature ventricular contraction

7. This is called _____.

bigeminy

8. The PVCs are (unifocal/multifocal). _____
_____

unifocal (they all have the same configuration)

9. When do the PVCs strike in relation to the T waves? _____
_____

Right after the T wave

10. Bigeminy might lead to _____
_____.

ventricular tachycardia or ventricular fibrillation

11. You would treat these ectopic beats with _____.

lidocaine

12. Sometimes bigeminy is a sign of _____ toxicity.

digitalis

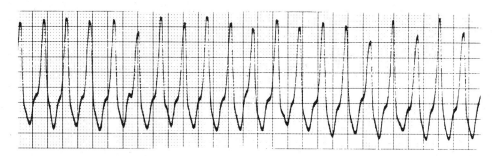

Figure 12.5. MR. V. T.

13. PVCs all in a row and at a rate of _____ per minute!

200 (20 PVCs in six seconds)

14. Run, don't walk, with a syringe of _____.

lidocaine

15. At any moment Mr. V.T. might develop _____ _____.

ventricular fibrillation

16. Bring the _____ to the bedside.

defibrillator

The alarm sounds and you see the ECG in Figure 12.6.

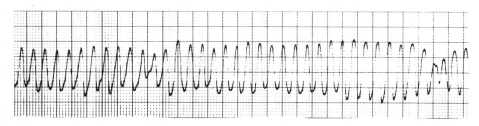

Figure 12.6. Ms. O. Lord.

17. The diagnosis of _____
seems likely, but you can't be sure.

extreme ventricular tachycardia

18. The first thing you would do is _____ the patient.

examine

19. You must find out if she is _____ _____ _____.   conscious or unconscious

20. She complains of marked shortness of breath. No wonder, her ventricular rate is nearly _____!   400 per minute

21. You would inject _____ instantly.   lidocaine

22. It doesn't work. She is not responding. What now? You would _____ the patient without delay.   defibrillate

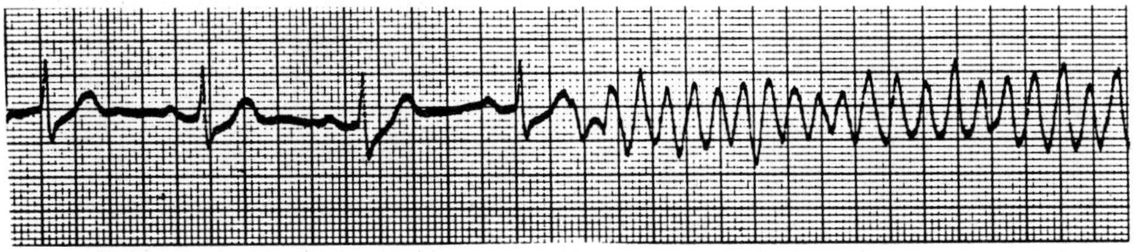

Figure 12.7. Mr. Enswell.

Analyze this ECG very carefully. It tells so much about the onset of ventricular arrhythmias.

23. The first four beats originate in the _____ _____.   SA node

24. They appear normal, except for _____ of the ST segments.   depression

25. Now look at the T wave of the 4th beat. It starts just as the first three did, and seems okay, *until* a _____ strikes on the downstroke of the wave.   PVC

26. This is called the _____-on-_____ phenomenon.   R   T

27. By striking during this phase of the cardiac cycle (called the vulnerable phase), the PVS caused the ventricle to fire repetitively and the patient developed _____ _____.   extreme ventricular tachycardia

28. Can you be sure of this diagnosis from the ECG above? _____   No

29. It might also be the beginning of _____ _____!   ventricular fibrillation

30. In either case, you wouldn't spend any more time looking at the monitor. You would go and _____ the patient.   examine

31. You find he is unconscious and has no pulses. Would you draw up 100-mg lidocaine and inject it? _____   No!

32. Waste no time. Use _____ _____ to terminate the arrhythmia.   precordial shock

I am happy to tell you that precordial shock was effective for this patient. He returned to normal sinus rhythm and recovered.

ACCELERATED IDIOVENTRICULAR RHYTHM *(pp. 209–211)*

Review 8

1. In ventricular tachycardia the rate is usually _____ to _____/minute.   140   250

2. Ventricular tachycardia is actually a series of consecutive _____.   PVCs

3. A series of PVCs at a slower rate, 50 to 100/minute, is called _____ _____ _____.   accelerated idioventricular rhythm

4. It is differentiated from ventricular tachycardia by its _____.   rate

5. Ventricular tachycardia usually starts and stops (gradually/abruptly).   abruptly

6. Accelerated idioventricular rhythm usually starts and stops (gradually/abruptly).   gradually

7. Incidentally, the inherent pacing rate of ventricular tissue is _____ to _____/ minute. | 25 40

8. When ventricular tissue fires at a rate of _____ to _____/minute, it is termed "accelerated." | 50 100

9. If the _____ nodal rate slows due to _____ or _____ toxicity, an accelerated ventricular pacemaker can take over. | SA ischemia digitalis

10. This (is/is not) a dangerous arrhythmia. | is not

11. Its only danger would be if it occurs together with ventricular _____. | tachycardia

12. The drug, _____, may be used to increase the SA nodal rate. | atropine

13. If the patient is receiving regular doses of _____, you would call the doctor before giving the next dose. | digitalis

VENTRICULAR FIBRILLATION: A FATAL ARRHYTHMIA *(pp. 212–216)*

This ECG pattern is one of the most awesome you will ever see: *ventricular fibrillation!*

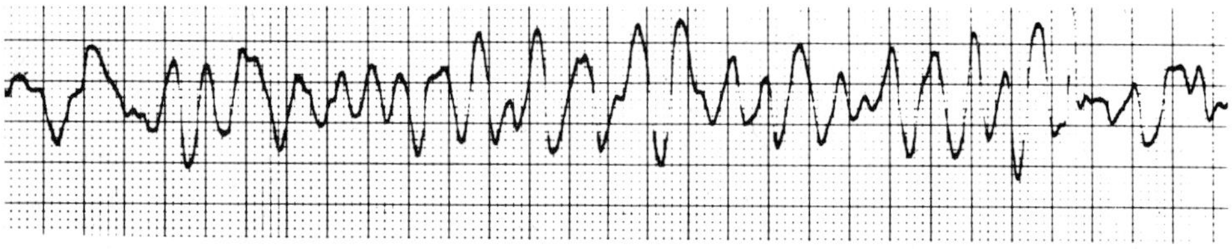

Figure 12.8

Review 9

1. In ventricular fibrillation the heart muscles merely _____. | twitch

2. The ventricles (do/do not) contract. | do not

3. The ventricles (do/do not) pump blood. | do not

4. Would you find any pulse in a patient with ventricular fibrillation? _____ | No

5. How would this patient appear? _____ or _____. | Unconscious convulsing

6. Ventricular fibrillation is probably caused by chaotic _____ activity in the ventricle. It is generally preceded by _____. | electrical PVCs

7. After an AMI the injured myocardium is thought to be extra-sensitive to _____ _____. | electrical stimulus

8. Also there may be multiple small waves of _____ leading to ventricular fibrillation. | re-entry

9. Most often ventricular fibrillation is caused by the R-on-T phenomena (a PVC hits the vulnerable phase at the time of the _____ wave). | T

10. The average time between the onset of ventricular fibrillation and death is about _____ _____. | three minutes

11. This means defibrillation must be accomplished within _____ _____. | three minutes

Okay, keep the above information in mind, and let's imagine that we are at the bedside of the patient whose monitor pattern shows ventricular fibrillation.

160

Review 10

1. Rule number one: Always treat the _____, not the monitor.

2. Check the patient. If he has ventricular fibrillation, you will find no peripheral _____.

3. You will hear no _____ _____ with a stethoscope. (And don't waste time running for a stethoscope if you haven't one hanging around your neck.)

4. You will find no _____ _____. (Again, I wouldn't waste time running for equipment; if other signs were positive, I wouldn't even waste time checking it.)

5. The patient will probably be _____.

6. The pupils soon (dilate/constrict).

7. The patient's color probably is _____.

8. He (may/may not) convulse.

9. What should you do? _____

Think of that! You must reach the bedside, diagnose by checking the patient as well as the monitor, and defibrillate him—all within three minutes. (Come back here, you don't have time to run for help!) It *can* be done, but don't pat yourself on the back until you can do it in less than two minutes. You may have to make some changes in the physical setup in your hospital to save time, and you will have to run some practice drills. But it is possible, and it's a tremendous thrill to succeed—*you have saved someone's life!*

Answers: patient / pulses / heart sounds / blood pressure / unconscious / dilate / cyanotic / may / Defibrillate him, STAT!

Treatment (pp. 214–215)

Review 11

1. The first step is _____ or _____ of the problem.

2. The monitor tips you off, but you actually confirm the diagnosis at the _____.

3. You will find that the patient is _____ and that he has no _____ _____.

4. The only treatment for ventricular fibrillation is _____. If there is any delay, start CPR.

5. Defibrillation should be performed within _____ minutes or less.

6. You should use the _____–_____ energy setting for defibrillation.

7. These patients all develop acidosis called _____ _____.

8. Lactic acidosis can be treated with _____ _____ IV.

9. After successful defibrillation, you must prevent _____.

10. The best prevention is continuous IV _____.

11. _____ may be used if lidocaine is ineffective.

Answers: recognition diagnosis / bedside / unconscious peripheral pulses / defibrillation / three / 200–360 J / lactic acidosis / sodium bicarbonate / recurrences / lidocaine / Bretylium

Nursing Responsibility *(p. 215)*

Read page 215 in *The Manual* very, very carefully. You won't have time to read it when ventricular fibrillation strikes.

Review 12

Now see if you can recall the first nine steps of the nursing role. I will start you off. (Don't go into details of the defibrillation process yet; we will do that in the next exercise.)

1. Monitor alarm sounds

2. _____

3. _____

4. _____

5. _____

6. _____

7. _____

8. _____

9. _____

    Check your answers with page 215 in *The Manual* and repeat this exercise until you can list all nine steps. Picture yourself doing each step as you list it.

Review 13

Now concentrate on the process of defibrillation as you would perform it. After you complete these statements, check your answers with the discussion that follows.

1. Before turning the machine on, spread _____ on the paddles.

2. Turn the defibrillator _____.

3. Set energy level at _____.

4. And be sure synchronizer is _____.

5. Place paddles on the chest so the current will go _____ the heart.

6. Hold the paddles _____ on the chest.

7. When discharging the shock, do not lean against the _____.

8. Be sure no one else touches the _____.

9. And do not touch the _____ yourself except through the paddles with insulated handles.

10. Let everybody know you are ready to deliver the shock by saying _____.

11. If you have successfully defibrillated the patient, the monitor should no longer show _____.

12. If you are successful, your patient's circulation returns: what three signs should you find? _____

    _____

    and _____.

13. Suppose you don't succeed, and the monitor still shows ventricular fibrillation; you would _____ again.

14. But after three unsuccessful shocks, you would stop, and start _____ STAT!

15. Patients with ventricular fibrillation will almost always develop _____ _____, and you will need _____ _____ to treat it.

16. If your patient is still in ventricular fibrillation and you are doing effective CPR and have sodium bicarbonate running in, then try _____ again.

Answers and Discussion

1. *Electrode paste or jelly.* Rub the paddles together to evenly spread the paste. DO THIS WITH THE DEFIBRILLATOR TURNED OFF, PLEASE! Instead of the paste, some hospitals use saline-soaked gauze pads. Place the pads on the chest and press the defibrillator paddles firmly over them. The pads must be wet, but not dripping; a trickle of saline running across the chest can conduct a spark and possibly burn the skin. The advantage of saline pads is that they don't leave a lot of slippery goop on the chest to interfere with cardiopulmonary resuscitation, should it be needed.

2, 3, and 4. Ready to go? Turn the defibrillator *ON,* set energy level at 200 J. Synchronizer must be *OFF.*

5. *Across* the heart. Do not put the paddles on the monitor electrodes or wires—you may defibrillate the monitor. When attaching the monitor electrodes it is wise to initially leave open space on the chest for defibrillation; nobody has time to reposition monitor leads before defibrillating a patient.

6. *Firmly.* Don't rock or tip them. If you do, you may produce a fireworks display and burn the patient in the process. Worse, the current may not go through to the heart.

7, 8, and 9. Three safety rules: nobody touches the *patient,* or the *bed,* or the *defibrillator cart.* Don't lean over and touch any of these yourself. If you are delivering the shock, it's up to you to ensure everyone else's safety. And if you work with some knuckleheaded doctor who insists he is going to continue with CPR or "bagging" (breathing) the patient while you shock, tell him that he must move away or you may have to defibrillate him, too.

10. Even if you must shout, be sure everyone knows when you are going to defibrillate. I don't care if you say, *"Fire!" "Shock!" "Ready—go!" Say something!*

11. *Fibrillation.* Sometimes the pattern after defibrillation isn't exactly normal, but if ventricular fibrillation has stopped and the patient's condition improves, don't defibrillate again; just hang in there.

12. The patient's *pulses* return; he has a measurable *blood pressure;* his *color* improves, *pupils constrict,* and, the greatest joy of all, he says, "Hey, watcha' do that for?"

13. *Defibrillate.* Increase energy level to 200 to 300 J. Maximum for third shock, 360 J.

14. *CPR*—before there's any chance of brain damage. How long have you spent defibrillating? Five minutes? Too long. Three minutes? That's more like it. Do CPR for a few minutes to circulate blood and oxygen to the brain, then defibrillate again if fibrillation continues. Remember, fibrillation does NOT circulate the blood; you must do that with CPR.

15. *Lactic acidosis* will occur; get the *sodium bicarbonate* going. One hint: if you must draw up sodium bicarbonate into a syringe, get the largest needle you can find. It may look clear in the vial, but it's as thick as pea soup when you try to draw it up.

16. *Defibrillation.* If you are circulating oxygen to the brain and counteracting lactic acidosis and he's still fibrillating—shock him again. Sometimes Bretylium or IV epinephrine is given to "strengthen" the fibrillation, and then defibrillation may be successful. With more than one nurse present, these things can be done almost simultaneously. Just don't shock your CPR givers and your IV helper—you need them!

Exercise 14

He has been in the CCU for two days and hasn't had any serious complications. Suddenly the alarm rings! You look at the monitor and see this:

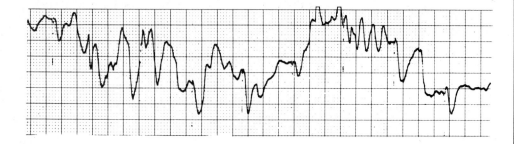

Figure 12.9. Mr. B. Ware.

No question about it—ventricular fibrillation. You grab the defibrillator and race to the bedside, not a second lost. You slop the electrode paste on and—STOP! Mr. Ware opens his eyes and protests, "Hey, what are ya doin'? What's goin' on?"

1. Mr. Ware (is/is not) in ventricular fibrillation.

           is not

2. The electrical pattern is probably an _____.

           artifact

3. The point is, always treat the _____ and not the _____!

           patient   monitor

Although the ECG looks like ventricular fibrillation, Mr. Ware would certainly *not* be alert and talking to you if this really were the problem. We are seeing an *artifact* on the monitor: Something has happened to the electrodes or the machine. Remember: treat the *patient,* not the *monitor.*

13

Disorders of Conduction
and Ventricular Asystole

CLASSIFICATION OF CONDUCTION DISORDERS

Review 1

One of the basic premises of medicine is that nearly everything has three names. The classification of conduction disorders is no exception. So hang in there, and let's see how you do.

1. A conduction disorder implies that the impulse originates _____, but that its conduction is _____ at some point thereafter.

    normally (in the SA node)
    blocked

2. Initially, the impulse can be blocked before it ever leaves the _____ _____.

    SA node

3. Or the impulse can make it into the atria where it can be blocked in the _____ tracts.

    internodal

4. These disorders would be classified as blocks in the _____ node or _____.

    SA   atria

5. Incidentally, you cannot differentiate these blocks from _____ _____ on an ECG.

    SA arrest

6. If an impulse that originated in the SA node makes it through the atria, it could be blocked in the _____ node, or in the area surrounding the node, called the _____ area.

    AV
    junctional

7. Because this area of blockage is between the atria and ventricles, we can call it an _____ block.

    atrioventricular

8. This area is a junction, or joining area, so we can substitute the phrase "_____ block."

    junctional

9. If the electrical impulse makes it through the junctional area, it has successfully passed *through* the _____ _____ _____ to its bifurcation.

    bundle of His

10. The impulse can still be blocked below the level of _____ of the bundle of His.

    bifurcation

11. Blocks below the bifurcation, because they are within the ventricles, can be termed _____ blocks.

intraventricular

12. More specifically, they may be hemiblocks or _____ blocks. (More on this later.)

fascicular

Review 2

This all may seem a little complicated, so let's try it in diagrammatic fashion. Label the following picture to see if you can visualize the areas where conduction blocks occur.

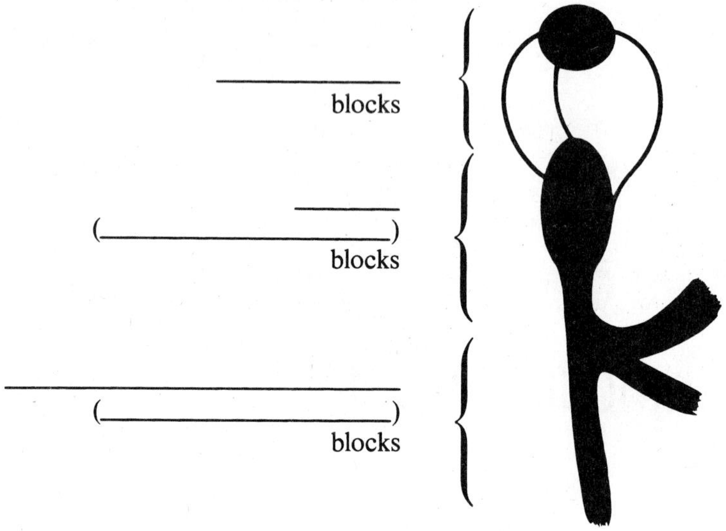

_____
blocks

(_____)
blocks

_____
(_____)
blocks

SA node

AV
(junctional)

Intraventricular
(subjunctional)

Figure 13.1

ATRIOVENTRICULAR (JUNCTIONAL) BLOCKS *(pp. 221–222)*

We will skip over SA node and atrial blocks because they really can't be differentiated from sinus arrest. In any event they are treated in the same fashion.

Atrioventricular (or junctional) blocks are divided into three classes. To picture them clearly, we need to use our imaginations. Suppose we think of the heart as being a very old-fashioned (no elevator), but very fancy, two-story apartment house. Access to the stairway between floors is controlled by a doorman, tottery old Mr. A. V. Node. The upper floor is called The Atria and the lower floor is called The Ventricles. People (electrical impulses) must go down a stairway to pass from The Atria to The Ventricles.

If Mr. A. V. Node is doing his job of opening the door properly as soon as an impulse arrives, it takes less than 0.20 seconds to travel from Atria to Ventricles. But A. V. Node sometimes slows down, and then it takes longer than 0.20 seconds for impulses to reach the Ventricles (first-degree heart block). At other times he takes a rest and won't open the door for each impulse that arrives. He may block every second or third or fourth impulse from reaching the Ventricles (second-degree heart block). Worst of all, A. V. Node may tire out and fall asleep. No impulses can then pass the nodal staircase—*all* are blocked (third-degree heart block).

Review 3

Keeping old Mr. A. V. Node in mind, try the following questions to see if you have the basic ideas.

1. First-, second-, and third-degree AV blocks are subdivisions of _____ (or _____) blocks.

atrioventricular
junctional

2. In first-degree AV block the impulse is _____, but it is eventually _____ to the ventricles.

delayed
conducted

3. In second-degree AV block _____, but not _____, impulses are _____.

some   all   blocked

4. In third-degree AV block _____ impulses are _____.

all   blocked

5. Thus, _____ impulses are conducted from atria to ventricles in third-degree block.

no

INTRAVENTRICULAR BLOCKS *(pp. 222–223)*

Say goodbye to Mr. A. V. Node because we are leaving his territory. Now we are going to consider blocks occurring *below* the level of bifurcation of the bundle of His.

Review 4

1. Do you know what bifurcation means? _____
   If not, look it up.

??
!!

2. Intraventricular blocks developing *after* an MI usually mean that there is _____ to the conduction pathways, probably in the interventricular _____ area.

injury
septal

3. Intraventricular blocks existing *before* an MI usually indicate a chronic _____ _____ of the bundle branches.

degeneration or
scarring

Review 5

Ready to work on the anatomy and physiology of the bundle branches?

1. Electrical conduction passes through the AV node to the _____ _____ _____.

bundle of
His

2. The bundle of His divides into two main branches. One of those branches is called the *right bundle branch* or _____. (initials)

RBB

3. The other branch is abbreviated as _____.

LBB

4. The LBB divides almost immediately into two branches. Another term for branches is _____.

fascicles

5. The fascicle serving the front portion of the heart would be called the _____ fascicle of the LBB.

anterior

6. The branch going to the back of the heart would be called the _____ _____ of the LBB.

posterior
fascicle

7. Thus, there is a total of _____ fascicles.

three (two from LBB, one
from RBB)

So far, so good. Now let's consider where blocks could occur in the bundle branches. Use the initials for your answers.

8. A block in the main right bundle branch is called an _____.

RBBB

9. A block in the main left bundle branch is called an _____.

LBBB

10. A block in the anterior fascicle of the LBB is called an _____.

LAH

11. The H in LAH stands for _____.

hemiblock

12. A block in the posterior fascicle of the LBB is called an _____.

LPH

13. Now suppose there is a block of the RBB plus one of the two left fascicles, you would call it a _____ _____.

bifascicular block (that's two
of the three branches)

14. Or (really bad) a block of all three branches below the bundle of His would be a _____ _____.

trifascicular block (all three
branches)

Review 6

If you are having trouble with any of the material on conduction blocks, or if you just want to make sure you know it, try the Mix and Match below and on the next page. Write the correct mixers in front of the matches.

MIXERS	MATCHES	
1. SA block	_____ block in right bundle branch	5
2. first-degree block	_____ block in anterior fascicle of left bundle branch	7
3. second-degree block	_____ AV node blocks *some* impulses	3
4. third-degree block	_____ block in SA node or atria	1
5. RBBB	_____ block in posterior fascicle of left bundle branch	8
6. LBBB	_____ AV node blocks all impulses	4
7. LAH	_____ block in all three bundle branch fascicles	10
8. LPH	_____ delay in conduction to ventricles	2
9. bifascicular block	_____ block in left main bundle branch	6
10. trifascicular block	_____ block in the right bundle branch plus one fascicle of left bundle branch	9

FIRST-DEGREE ATRIOVENTRICULAR HEART BLOCK *(pp. 224–226)*

Review 7

We haven't tried any true or false questions for a while, so let's try some. Note whether the statements below are true or false. Remember, they all refer to first-degree AV block.

_____	1. Does not reduce hemodynamic efficiency of the heart.	T
_____	2. Delayed conduction shows in the P–R interval.	T
_____	3. Vagal overactivity can be a cause.	T
_____	4. Does affect rate or rhythm.	F
_____	5. P–R interval longer than 0.28 is more dangerous.	T
_____	6. P–R interval is 0.21 or greater.	T
_____	7. Usually treat only if it is progressive or extreme.	T
_____	8. Atropine is not a treatment.	F
_____	9. Antiarrhythmic drugs can be a cause.	T
_____	10. Impulses are blocked in the AV node.	F
_____	11. Diagnosis is by ECG.	T
_____	12. Atropine 0.1 to 0.5 mg IV is standard treatment.	F
_____	13. Prepare for transvenous pacing if progressive.	T
_____	14. Notify doctor if P–R is greater than 0.28.	T
_____	15. Digitalis is not a possible cause.	F
_____	16. Caused by ischemia of the AV node.	T
_____	17. Patient is aware of sensation of irregularity.	F
_____	18. May warn of impending second- or third-degree block.	T

_____	19. Is a serious arrhythmia in its own right.	F
_____	20. Don't begin treatment unless P–R is 0.36 or greater.	F
_____	21. Most commonly seen in inferior AMIs.	T

SECOND-DEGREE ATRIOVENTRICULAR BLOCK

Mobitz Type I (Wenckebach) Block *(pp. 227–230)*
Review 8

Second-degree heart block—this is where our doorman, AV Node, blocks some but not all conduction between the atria and ventricles. Sometimes the old gentleman tries hard to keep up with his job. However, he tires out and takes longer to allow each impulse through the conduction stairway. Finally, he has to take a brief rest and, as a result, one impulse is blocked from reaching the ventricles. He then feels refreshed and goes back to work, starting the cycle all over again. How do we know this about AV Node's behavior? The ECG shows us a series of increasingly prolonged P–R intervals until one P wave is not followed by a QRS. After the blocked beat, the pattern repeats itself.

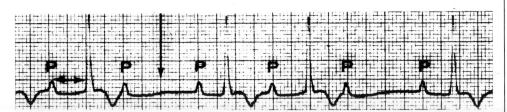

Figure 13.2. This conduction disturbance is called Wenckebach (wink-key-bok) type second-degree block or Mobitz Type I.

1. In Mobitz Type I blocks you will find (more/fewer) P waves than QRSs. — more
2. The P–R interval will (increase/decrease) with each beat. — increase
3. Finally, an impulse (is/is not) conducted. — is not
4. The ventricular rhythm (will/will not) be regular. — will not
5. The basic pacemaker is the _____ _____. — SA node
6. The problem lies in the _____ _____. — AV node
7. There is a (progressive/constant) slowing of conduction through the AV node. — progressive
8. This is the (mildest/severest) form of second-degree heart block. — mildest
9. Mobitz Type I (can/cannot) progress to third-degree block. — can
10. If the heart rate drops below 50, treatment with _____ is indicated. — isoproterenol
11. What drugs would you withhold until further orders? _____ _____ — digitalis quinidine procainamide propranolol

SECOND-DEGREE ATRIOVENTRICULAR HEART BLOCK *(pp. 231–233)*
Mobitz Type II Block
Review 9

You have just learned that Mobitz Type I is a form of second-degree block in which the P–R interval varies. Now we are going to compare this to second-degree block with a constant P–R but with some missing (blocked) QRSs.

1. Mobitz Type I is caused by an injury to the _____ _____.

   AV node

2. In Type II Mobitz the block is (below/above) the AV junction; this is termed a _____ block. This is (less/much more) serious.

   below
   subjunction   much more

3. You may see a 2:1 type second-degree block; however, the block can be _____ or _____ etc.

   3:1
   4:1

4. Type II may occur with _____ or _____ AMIs.

   anterior   anteroseptal

5. There are (more/fewer) P waves than QRSs.

   more

6. In 2:1 block there are _____ P waves for each QRS.

   two

7. In 3:1 block there are _____ P waves for each QRS.

   three

8. 3:1 block (is/is not) the same as third-degree heart block.

   is not

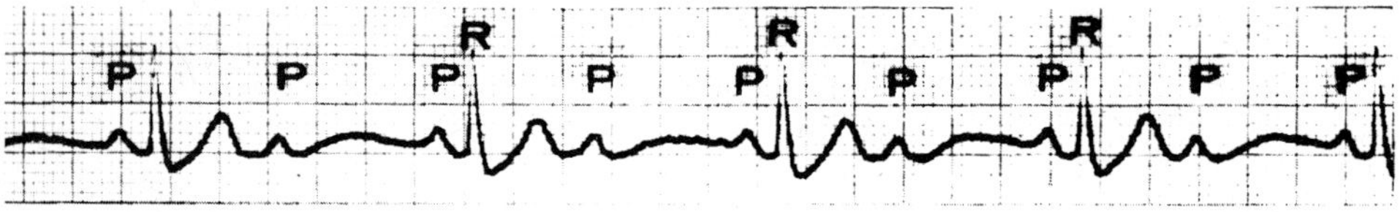

Figure 13.3

Review 10

The following questions relate to second-degree block with a constant P–R.

1. The QRS complexes occur (regularly/irregularly) when the block is constant.

   regularly

2. The P waves occur (regularly/irregularly).

   regularly

3. The P–R interval of the beats that are conducted (is/is not) constant.

   is

4. The degree of block may change. (True/False)

   True

5. Because the block is below the junction, a junctional pacemaker (can/cannot) take over; only _____ pacemakers are left.

   cannot
   ventricular

6. Type II block is usually associated with (anterior/posterior) MIs.

   anterior

7. The drug _____ is not recommended as it does not decrease the degree of _____.

   atropine
   block

8. The more blocked beats, the more serious the block. (True/False)

   True

9. Type II blocks (are/are not) stable.

   are not

10. Type II blocks can be a forerunner of _____-_____ _____ or ventricular _____.

   third-degree block (complete)
   standstill

THIRD-DEGREE (COMPLETE) ATRIOVENTRICULAR HEART BLOCK (pp. 234–238)
Review 11

In third-degree block, old Mr. AV Node has had it. No impulses can reach the ventricle. The sinus impulses may continue to bombard the AV node regularly, but none of them is conducted to the ventricles. This is the condition we feared in patients with first- and second-degree heart block. This is what we had hoped to prevent. We now have a critical problem.

1. In third-degree block the atria are paced by the _____ _____.

   SA node

2. Thus, we see normal _____ waves.

   P

3. (Some/All) of the P waves are blocked.

   All

4. Another name for third-degree block is _____ heart block.

complete

5. In acute MI, this block is usually caused by _____ damage of the junctional area or lower conduction system.

ischemic

6. Since none of the atrial impulses reach the ventricles, what causes the ventricles to contract? _____ _____

Either a junctional or a ventricular pacemaker.

7. If the block occurs (above/below) the bifurcation of the bundle of _____, a junctional pacemaker may take over.

above   His

8. Junctional escape pacemakers can cause ventricular conduction at a rate of _____ to _____ per minute.

40
60

9. What will the atrial rate be? _____.

Whatever the SA node is doing

10. However, the block may occur *below* the _____ of the bundle of His, then the ventricular rate would probably be _____ to _____ per minute.

bifurcation
30   40

11. The atrial rate will be (faster than/slower than/the same as) the ventricular rate, whether the block is above or below the bifurcation.

faster than

12. There (is/is not) a relationship between atrial and ventricular conductions.

is not

13. As a result, the P–R interval (is/is not) constant.

is not

14. There (is/is not) a relationship between P waves and QRSs.

is not

15. You might say the atria and ventricles are divorced; the medical term for this is _____ _____.

atrioventricular dissociation

16. The independent ventricular pacemaker (is/is not) dependable.

is not

17. Effective conductions (may/may not) cease at any moment.

may

18. This would cause a lethal arrhythmia: _____ _____.

ventricular standstill

19. In addition, there is the threat of a faster ventricular focus taking over and causing _____ _____.

ventricular tachycardia or ventricular fibrillation

20. The ventricular rate (can/cannot) increase to meet circulatory demands.

cannot

21. Thus, the patient often has inadequate _____ _____.

cardiac output

22. What cerebral symptoms might you expect in a patient with third-degree heart block? _____, _____, _____, _____.

confusion   lightheadedness
fainting   convulsions

23. This ventricular rate below 40 that cannot _____ with activity (is/is not) adequate.

increase   is not

24. These patients may also develop symptoms of _____ _____ _____.

left ventricular
    failure

25. Complete heart block (is/is not) an extremely dangerous arrhythmia.

is

Review 12

Imagine you have just admitted a patient with complete heart block; treatment has not yet been started.

1. Your patient may suddenly _____ or _____.

faint   convulse

2. The best overall treatment for complete heart block is _____ _____.

transvenous pacing

3. Ideally, a transvenous pacing catheter should be inserted _____ third-degree begins.

before

4. A pacing catheter should be left in place at least _____ days after NSR is reestablished.

five

171

5. Unfortunately, in this patient, none is in place; therefore you should (get ready/wait for an order) for insertion of a pacing catheter.

get ready

6. One drug that may help in the meantime is _____.

Isuprel

7. Very slow ventricular rates can allow _____ and _____ _____ to occur.

PVCs ventricular fibrillation

8. If third-degree heart block does not subside, but becomes permanent, it can be treated with a permanent _____.

pacemaker

Review 13

These questions also refer to the patient in complete heart block.

1. First, you must _____ or _____ the arrhythmia and document or record it.

identify diagnose

2. When would you call the doctor? _____

STAT

3. What drug would you have ready? _____

Isoproterenol

4. The order might be for _____ mg Isuprel in _____ cc dextrose in water IV.

1   250

5. You would know that the drug should be given very _____.

slowly

6. You would watch the monitor for _____ _____.

ectopic beats

7. This patient may suddenly go into ventricular _____.

fibrillation

8. So you would bring the _____ to the bedside.

defibrillator

9. You would also bring a syringe of 100 mg _____ (ie, _____) to the bedside.

lidocaine xylocaine

10. Where would you put the crash cart? _____

At the bedside.

11. How does the patient feel about all this activity? _____

Scared!

Take a moment to consider this patient. He is terrified. Can you screen some of this awesome equipment, yet have it instantly ready? Can you be calm and matter-of-fact? Know where things are; know what you need. Be prepared. Then you can reassure this patient honestly and convincingly that everything possible is being done. Is it important to talk to this patient? Many patients describe a "fading away" and an enclosing blackness. They say the nurse's voice was their only reassurance.

I remember particularly a woman with third-degree heart block whose transvenous pacemaker failed in the middle of the night. Her ventricular rate fell to about 35 per minute. And then she went into ventricular fibrillation. After we defibrillated her, she developed ventricular standstill. External pacing was only partially successful and she found it extremely painful. So we alternately used cardiopulmonary resuscitation, defibrillation, and external pacing until the doctor arrived and inserted a new pacing catheter. Later, before she went home, she told us, "It was the sound of your voice that pulled me through. I'd climb up out of a dark pit and there'd be a horrible crushing on my chest. Then I'd hear a beautiful voice saying: 'Hang on, Mary, we won't let you die. Keep trying just a little bit longer.' And so I kept trying."

There are excellent examples of third-degree heart block shown on pages 235–236 of *The Manual.* Measure out P–P and R–R intervals with your scrap paper. Prove to yourself that the atria and ventricles are divorced totally and completely. Measure the P–R intervals and prove that they are never constant.

MONITOR PRACTICE

Review 14

Okay, let's set up our mythical CCU. You already have three patients and you are going to admit Mr. Percival Long and Mr. Adam Stokes. Let's check their monitors and answer some questions.

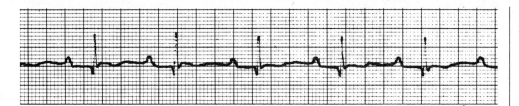

Figure 13.4. Mr. Percival Long.

This is an admission rhythm strip.

1. What is the ventricular rate? _____

70 per minute

2. Are the P waves normal? _____

Yes

3. Are the QRS complexes normal? _____

Yes

4. He is in _____ _____ rhythm.

normal sinus

5. Then what's the problem? _____
_____
_____.

The P–R interval is prolonged to 0.28 seconds. This is first-degree heart block.

6. What would you watch for in this patient? _____.

Signs of advancing heart block

7. Is any treatment necessary now? _____

No

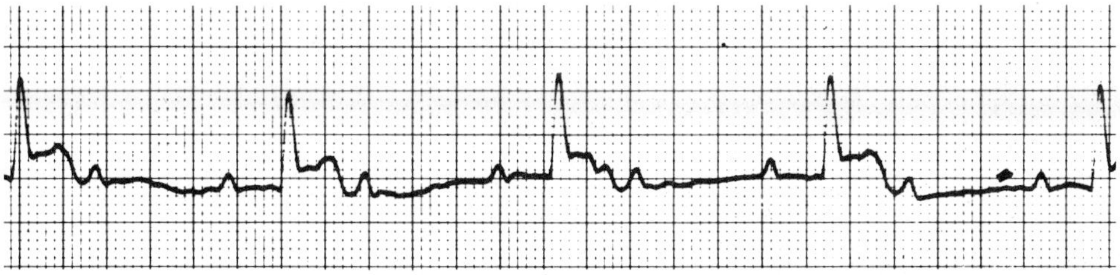

Figure 13.5. Mr. Kon Fuze.

Confused? Well let's see if we can make some sense out of this ECG.

1. Find the R waves. What is the ventriculr rate? _____

50 per minute

2. Now pick out the P waves. Don't let that step-stool after the R waves fool you—it's an elevated _____ segment.

ST

3. How many P waves are there in this six-second strip? _____

10

4. This means the atrial rate is _____ per minute.

100 (10 × 10)

5. We now know the atrial rate is faster than the ventricular rate. There are _____ P waves for each _____ complex.

two
QRS

6. This tells us that every other P wave is _____, and not conducted.

blocked

7. The P–R interval of the conducted beats is (constant/inconstant).

constant

8. The P–R interval of the conducted beats is _____ seconds.

0.28

9. The interpretation of this ECG is _____-_____ heart block with _____ block.

second-degree
2:1

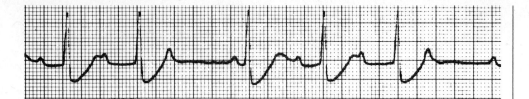

Figure 13.6. Mr. W. Bokman.

1. Is the rhythm regular? _____

No

2. What is the ventricular rate? _____

70 per minute

3. Study the first three beats on the strip. What do you notice? _____
_____.

The P–R interval increases with each beat

4. This means there is an increasing _____ in conducton through the AV node, until a beat is _____.

delay
blocked

5. This is a form of _____-degree heart block.

second

6. It is called _____ Type I block.

Mobitz

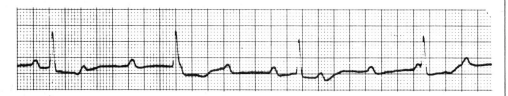

Figure 13.7. Ms. D. D.

She's in trouble, and we have to act quickly.

1. Her ventricular rate is only _____ per minute.

40

2. Measure out her P waves. Use a scrap paper and mark the first three P waves, then keep moving the marks across the strip. Are the P waves regular? _____. Did you find the fourth and ninth P waves hidden in or near the QRS complexes?

Yes (the P waves are regular)

3. What is the atrial rate? _____ per minute.

100 (10 P waves in 6 seconds × 10 = 100)

4. Is there any relationship between the P waves and QRS complexes? _____

No

5. Are the P–R intervals as constant as Mr. Kon Fuze's? _____
_____

No (The P–R intervals are *not* constant).

6. Ms. DD's atria and ventricles are divorced. She has developed _____
_____.

third-degree (complete) heart block

7. The slow ventricular rate is very dangerous because the cardiac output cannot be _____.

maintained

8. There is also a threat of _____ _____ developing.

ventricular fibrillation or ventricular standstill

9. What is the most dependable treatment for this problem? _____
_____ _____.

transvenous cardiac pacing

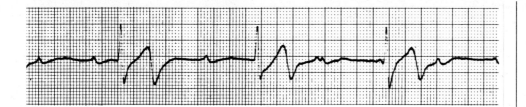

Figure 13.8. Mr. Adam Stokes.

This patient is unconscious when you admit him. You connect the monitor to this cold, clammy man and what do you see! (Can you imagine how you would feel?)

1. The ventricular rate is just _____ per minute.	30
2. The reason he's unconscious is that cerebral _____ _____ is inadequate.	blood flow (perfusion)
3. Are the atria beating faster than the ventricles? _____	Yes
4. Are the P–R intervals constant? _____	No
5. The ECG diagnosis is _____ _____ _____ .	complete heart block
6. As soon as you see this pattern, you would _____ !	call the doctor STAT
7. He is likely to order _____ IV until he gets there.	isoproterenol (Isuprel)
8. While he is on his way, you would prepare for _____ _____ _____ .	transvenous cardiac pacing

INTRAVENTRICULAR BLOCKS (BUNDLE-BRANCH BLOCKS) *(pp. 239–241)*

Are you sure of where we are? Just for orientation's sake, we are studying blocks *below* the AV junctional area, eg, bundle-branch blocks. Since bundle-branch blocks imply that something is wrong with the conduction pathway, let's start with a brief review of electrical conduction through the heart and then move on to the BBB (bundle-branch blocks).

Review 15

1. In first-, second-, or third-degree blocks, the conduction disturbance is in or near the _____ _____ .	AV node
2. In bundle branch blocks (BBB), conduction is normal through the AV node. (True/False)	True
3. The problem arises below the bifurcation of the _____ _____ _____ .	bundle of His
4. The block is in either the _____ bundle branch or _____ bundle branch of the bundle of His.	left right
5. This results in delayed activation of either the _____ or _____ ventricle, depending on which branch is blocked.	left right
6. If the right bundle branch is blocked, the right ventricle is stimulated through the _____ _____ .	interventricular septum
7. Consequently, the right ventricle would be stimulated (before/after) the left ventricle.	after
8. The time for both ventricles to be activated would be (longer/shorter) than normal.	longer
9. This delay is shown in the (PR/QRS) portion of the cycle.	QRS
10. The characteristic ECG finding of BBB is a prolonged _____ complex.	QRS
11. *Prolonged* means over _____ seconds in duration.	0.12

12. BBB may be (acute/chronic/both). | both

13. Chronic BBB is usually due to _____ _____ _____ of the bundle branches. | degeneration or scarring

14. Acute BBB develops as a complication of _____ _____. | acute MI

15. Acute BBB suggests that the _____ _____ has been injured. | interventricular septum

16. Prognosis in acute BBB is (better/worse) than in chronic BBB. | worse

Review 16

Use Figure 13.9 to help you understand the dangers of BBB.

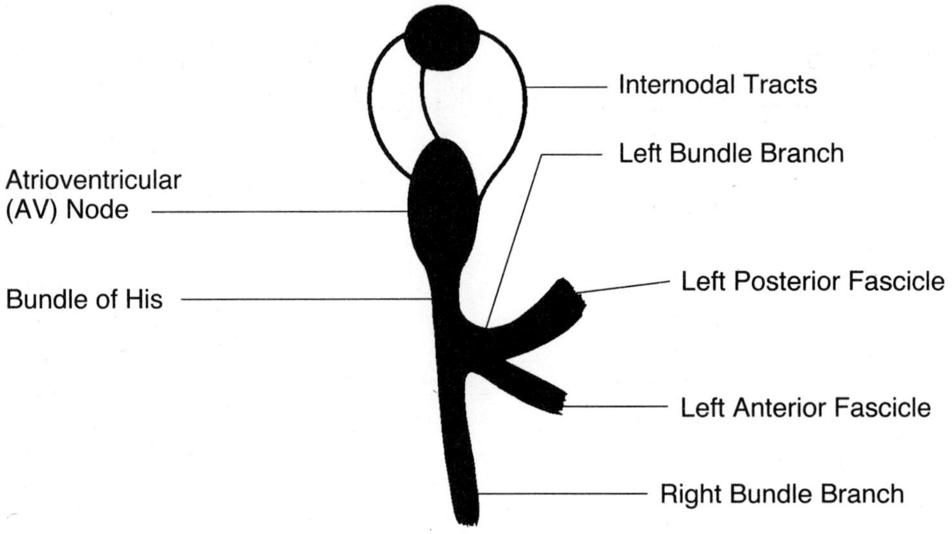

Figure 13.9

1. An acute block of more than one fascicle (is/is not) considered very dangerous. | is

2. A block of the _____ bundle branch obscures the diagnosis of MI. | left

3. Blocks of _____ fascicles are more dangerous than blocks of one pathway. | 2

4. If three pathways are blocked, _____ _____ may result. | ventricular standstill

5. Any degree of acute BBB indicates myocardial _____, especially of the _____ _____ area. | damage interventricular septal

Review 17

Mr. M. I. has been in the CCU for two days. Except for occasional PVCs, no other arrhythmias have occurred. The QRS complexes have been 0.08 seconds. Today you notice that the QRS has widened to 0.14 seconds. The heart rate is 70 beats per minute and you can identify P waves before each QRS complex.

1. What is the most likely diagnosis? _____ _____. | A bundle branch block has developed

2. How do you know that the wide QRS complexes aren't PVCs? _____ _____. | P waves are seen before each complex

3. Can you tell from the monitor if this is an RBBB or LBBB? _____ | No

4. How can you make sure? _____. | Take a 12-lead ECG

5. Can you tell from the monitor how many fascicles are involved? _____ | No

6. How can you tell? _____ | With a 12-lead ECG

7. Should you call the doctor? _____

      Yes

8. Why? _____
_____.

      Because this may be a warning of complete heart block or ventricular standstill

9. What treatment is likely to be used? _____
_____.

      Insertion of transvenous pacemaker

10. Overdose of _____ might possibly cause BBB.

      quinidine

VENTRICULAR ASYSTOLE: A FATAL ARRHYTHMIA *(pp. 242–246)*

We have already discussed ventricular fibrillation. Now we come to the other sudden death arrhythmia—ventricular asystole (eg, "Hey, look at the monitor. He's in asystole!"). Without a monitor, you can't tell the difference between the two sudden death arrhythmias. The circulation stops in both circumstances. And not so long ago, before we had coronary care units, the treatment was identical; at least we can save lives after ventricular fibrillation. But what about ventricular asystole? Well, the picture here isn't as bright. Most patients who develop ventricular asystole still die. But "most" doesn't mean *all,* and there is always a chance. With effective CPR we can maintain adequate circulation and hope that with pacing or drugs the doctor may be able to reverse this sudden death process.

Review 18

1. Without a monitor, or ECG, you (can/cannot) differentiate between ventricular fibrillation and ventricular asystole.

      cannot

2. Outside the CCU, any condition resulting in no circulation is termed _____ _____.

      cardiac
        arrest

3. The terms ventricular standstill, ventricular asystole, and cardiac arrest are used interchangeably. (True/False)

      True

4. In CCU the two preferred terms (of these four: ventricular standstill, ventricular fibrillation, ventricular asystole, cardiac arrest) are: _____ _____, and _____ _____.

      ventricular asystole
      ventricular fibrillation

5. Ventricular aystole may rarely occur as a primary electrical failure, most often it is a terminal arrhythmia in advanced _____ _____, (ie, _____ _____, or left ventricular _____.)

      heart failure   cardiogenic
        shock   failure

6. Sinus, atrial, or junctional impulses may continue but they are all _____ in ventricular asystole.

      blocked

7. If no ventricular pacemaker takes over, then _____ _____ occurs.

      ventricular asystole

8. In most cases, you will have seen some form of _____ block, usually _____, before asystole occurs.

      intraventricular
      bifascicular

9. In the dying patient, the electrical conductivity is depressed because of _____, _____ and _____ imbalance.

      hypoxia
      acidosis   electrolyte

10. In the dying heart, the electrical impulses may not cause contractions (although there may be weak, ineffectual contractions). This is called _____-_____ _____.

      electro-mechanical
        dissociation

12. (Ventricular asystole, ventricular fibrillation) is the most dreaded and dangerous of all arrhythmias.

      ventricular asystole

13. The only successful "treatment" is _____.

      prevention

14

Electrocardiographic Diagnosis of Myocardial Infarction, Injury, and Ischemia

Have you ever listened in as an ICCU nurse and a doctor studied a 12-lead ECG? "Look—there—and there. It's anterior!" "Right! And there—see that?"

No longer will you have to feel like Alice or Alex in Wonderland. You are going to be able to diagnose AMIs on a 12-lead ECG.

We have spent so much time on arrhythmias and conduction disorders that maybe you should go back and review Chapter 8. That's a foundation you are really going to need now. Then read page 251 in *The Manual*.

Review 1

Match the terms, A through D, to the statements.

TERMS

A. 12-lead ECG   B PET

C. Thallium scan   D Cardiac monitor

STATEMENTS

1. Measures extent of myocardial perfusion. _____   C

2. Identify arrhythmias. _____   D

3. Diagnose ischemia, injury, necrosis. _____   A

4. Thrombolysis started only after diagnosis with this. _____   A

5. Measure cellular metabolism. _____   B

6. Least expensive, safest. _____   A

DIAGNOSIS OF ACUTE MYOCARDIAL INFARCTION (*pp. 251–255*)

Review 2

1. The three zones of an acute MI are:
   Zone 1: _____, Zone 2: _____, Zone 3: _____.
   (Memorize these.)

   necrosis   injury   ischemia

2. The most severely damaged is zone _____, which is the zone of _____.

   1   necrosis

3. This shows on an ECG by changes in the (Q/ST/T) wave.

   Q

4. What are the changes? _____

   Deep, wide Q

5. Can you explain this? _____
   _____
   _____.

   ?

6. Let's try. The electrode is looking through a "window" of (dead/active) muscle. So it records electrical activity going (away from/toward) it. This activity is actually the first part of the _____ depolarizing. (Remember, a force going away from an electrode records as (negative/positive) on the ECG.

   dead
   away from
   septum
   negative

7. The Q waves of an acute MI occur after an MI (within an hour/within days/both/neither).

   both

8. Zone 2 of an acute MI is the area of _____.

   injury

9. Zone 2 shows on an ECG by changes in the (Q/ST/T).

   ST

10. The ST segment may be (elevated/depressed/both/neither).

    both

11. If the ECG lead faces the injured area, the ST will be _____.

    elevated

12. Depressed STs are also called _____ changes.

    reciprocal

13. Elevated STs are convex and sometimes called a _____ ST.

    coved

14. Coved STs show in leads (facing/away from) the injury.

    facing

15. Zone 3 of an MI is the area of _____.

    ischemia

16. Zone 3 shows on an ECG by changes in the (Q/ST/T).

    T

17. The T waves may be _____ and sharply _____.

    inverted   pointed

18. T wave changes (may/may not) be caused by things other than an MI.

    may

LOCALIZATION OF MYOCARDIAL INFARCTION (*pp. 255–258*)

Review 3

1. With an acute transmural MI, all three zones (may/may not) be seen on the ECG.

   may

2. So on an ECG you might find changes in _____, _____, and _____ waves.

   Q   ST   T

3. Do all three changes need to be present for the diagnosis of an MI? _____

   no

4. The ECG can tell you if the MI is an anterior, posterior, or inferior MI. (True/False)

   True

5. Why does it matter to you where the MI is located? _____
   _____

   Prognosis and complications correlate with the site.

6. Once again, the acute MI ECG pattern consists of _____,
   _____, and _____. (Memorize this—you will use it later in "diagnosing" MIs.)

   deep Q waves
   elevated ST segments
   inverted T waves

WHERE'S THE MYOCARDIAL INFARCTION?
Review 4

One of the favorite games in CCU is called "Where's His MI?" It's a thrill to "diagnose" a 12-lead ECG and find out the cardiologist's diagnosis agrees with yours! It takes lots of practice. To begin with, read pages 255–258 in *The Manual,* very carefully. Review 4 puts the material into a handy chart. Choose your answers from those given below. I suggest you photocopy the blank chart for extra practice. When you know the answer on the chart, then practice using the chart with real 12-lead ECGs and look for the changes in the leads specified.

Choices for answers in Review 4.

Characteristis and Complications Choices:

Higher incidence of heart block

Higher death rate

Higher incidence of pump failure

More frequently involves AV node

Involves larger pump mass

Electrocardiographic Changes:

(Choices include all ECG leads)

Leads I, II, III

aVL, aVF, aVR

V1-V6

ANTERIOR MI	INFERIOR MI
Characteristics and Complications	
1. _____	1. _____
2. _____	2. _____
3. _____	
Electrocardiographic Changes	
Acute MI pattern	*Acute MI pattern*
1. Extensive Anterior MI:	1. Inferior MI:
_____	_____
_____	_____
_____	_____
2. Anteroseptal MI:	2. Inferolateral MI:
_____	* _____
_____	_____
_____	_____
3. Anterolateral MI:	_____
_____	* _____
_____	* _____
_____	* = ST, T changes

ANTERIOR MI	INFERIOR MI
Characteristics and Complications	
1. Higher death rate	1. Higher incidence of heart block
2. Involves larger muscle mass	2. More frequently involves AV node
3. Higher incidence of pump failure	
Electrocardiographic Changes	
Acute MI pattern	*Acute MI pattern*
1. Extensive Anterior MI: Lead I aVL all V leads	1. Inferior MI: Lead II Lead III aVF
2. Anteroseptal MI: Lead I aVL V1–V4	2. Inferolateral MI: *Lead I Lead II Lead III aVF *aVL *V5–V6
3. Anterolateral MI: Lead I aVL V4–V6	* = ST, T changes

STAGES OF MYOCARDIAL INFARCTION *(pp. 258–266)*

Review 5

1. In Review 4 we learned the acute MI patterns in specific ECG leads that help us identify the _____ of an MI.

   location

2. The 12-lead ECG also shows the stages of _____ of an MI.

   healing

3. Three stages shown by the ECG are _____, _____, and _____.

   acute   recent   old

4. As you know, the acute MI pattern is _____, _____ _____, _____.

   deep Q waves   elevated STs   inverted T waves

5. When _____ and _____ return to normal (or stabilize), the MI is in the recent stage.

   ST   T

6. The "old" MI retains the _____ changes.

   Q

7. Pathological Q waves are wider than _____ second and deeper than _____ mm.

   0.04   4

NON–Q-WAVE MYOCARDIAL INFARCTION *(p. 266)*

Review 6

1. A nontransmural MI (does/does not) extend clear through the myocardium.

   does not

2. Nontransmural MIs produce only small patchy areas of _____ in the muscle.

   necrosis

3. Thus, the necrosis pattern of zone I, the _____ wave changes, are not found in the ECGs. | Q

4. Sometimes the only ECG change will be in the _____. | T

5. So nontransmural MIs may be called _____ _____ infarctions. | T wave

6. Anterior nontransmural ECG changes occur in leads _____, _____, and _____ _____ _____. | I aVL all V leads

7. Inferior nontransmural ECG changes occur in leads _____, _____, and _____. | II III aVF

8. The above are the same as in transmural MIs (see Review 4). (True/False) | True

9. T wave changes can occur for reasons other than an MI. (True/False) | True

10. Old nontransmural MIs can be identified by ECG changes. (True/False) | False

TRANSIENT MYOCARDIAL ISCHEMIA (ANGINA PECTORIS) *(pp. 266–271)*

Review 7

1. The underlying cause of angina pectoris is a transient _____ ischemia. | subendocardial

2. Ischemia of angina shows in _____ depression (*not* elevation), and sometimes in _____ wave changes. | ST T

3. This (is/is not) the same as the zones of injury change in acute MIs. (See Fig. 14–25 in *The Manual* to see why.) | is not

4. Variant angina pectoris, also called _____ involves pain (at rest/during exertion). | Prinzmetal's at rest

5. The underlying cause of variant angina is _____ _____ _____ which causes _____ ischemia. | coronary artery spasm subepicardial

6. This causes _____ segment (elevation/depression) on the ECG. | ST elevation

7. Can you differentiate between stable angina pectoris and variant angina on the ECG? (See Questions 2 and 6.) | Yes

8. After a period of variant angina, the ECG changes should promptly return to normal (the baseline). (True/False) | True

9. Failure to return to normal probably indicates _____ _____. | an acute MI, not just angina

ELECTROCARDIOGRAPHIC CHANGES WITH EXERCISE (STRESS) TESTING *(pp. 272–274)*

Review 8

1. Stress testing may be done to confirm the diagnosis of _____. | angina

2. Exercise is used to increase the myocardial _____ demand. | oxygen

3. ECGs taken before, during, and after exercise show myocardial _____ during exercise if the test is positive. | ischemia

4. This is shown by _____ _____ on the ECG. | ST depression

5. Stress testing (is/is not) entirely reliable. | is not

15

Cardiac Pacemakers

Sometimes the heart's electrical system is injured after an acute myocardial infarction and an artificial pacemaker is needed to keep the heart beating. In a sense, a pacemaker is a battery. It sends current to the heart by way of wires called catheter electrodes. Sounds simple, doesn't it? Let's keep it that way.

Review 1

1. Normally the ventricles contract in response to _____ stimuli originating within the heart.

   electrical

2. External electrical stimulus can also be used to make the ventricles _____.

   contract

3. This can be done with a _____.

   pacemaker

4. Pacemaker impulses are generated by a _____.

   battery

5. Pacemakers can be used if the _____ _____ of the heart fails to conduct impulses or they can be used to prevent or control _____.

   electrical system
   tachyarrhythmias

6. If the heart's pacing rate is too slow, _____ _____ can take over and cause tachyarrhythmias.

   ectopic foci

7. If the heart can be paced at a (slower/faster) rate the ectopic focus can be suppressed; this is called _____.

   faster
   overdriving

8. You would prefer a (transvenous/transcutaneous) pacemaker if possible. (Especially if you are the patient!)

   transvenous

9. In an emergency if there isn't time to insert a transvenous pacemaker, _____ pacing can be lifesaving.

   transcutaneous

10. There are three types of pacing: _____, temporary _____, and permanent _____.

    transcutaneous transvenous
    implanted

185

TRANSCUTANEOUS PACEMAKER *(p. 275)*

Review 2

1. Transcutaneous pacing can be used if the myocardium can still _____, but there are problems with impulse _____ or _____.

   contract
   formation   conduction

2. Two conducting _____ (6 to 8 inches) are applied, one to the _____ chest and one to the _____ chest and connected to the pacemaker control box.

   electrodes
   anterior   posterior

3. The anterior electrode goes below the _____ _____ of a female and the posterior one goes on the upper _____, _____ of the spine.

   left breast
   back   left

4. Set the pacing rate _____ to _____ beats per minute higher than the patient's intrinsic rate.

   10   20

5. If the patient is in asystole, set the rate at _____.

   60

6. The energy output (measured in _____) can be increased until _____ is obtained.

   joules   capture

TEMPORARY TRANSVENOUS PACEMAKER *(pp. 276–287)*

Review 3

1. A conduction disturbance may be temporary, eg, after an acute _____ MI, and temporary pacing may be needed.

   inferior

2. Ventricular asystole can result from heart blocks, especially _____ or _____-_____ heart block, or _____-_____ _____ of more than one _____.

   second-
   third-degree   bundle-branch
      block   fascicle

3. A transvenous pacemaker should be inserted (before/after) trouble develops.

   before

4. The primary purpose of transvenous pacing is to (detect/prevent/treat) ventricular asystole.

   prevent

5. Transvenous pacing is most often used to treat advancing forms of _____ _____.

   heart
      block

6. It can also be used to treat _____.

   bradycardias

7. With extreme bradycardias, premature ventricular contractions are (more likely/less likely) to occur.

   more likely

8. By (increasing/decreasing) the heart rate with a pacemaker, these PVCs may be eliminated.

   increasing

9. This is called _____ the heart.

   overdriving

10. The electrodes are placed in contact with the (endocardium/epicardium) and can be positioned to stimulate the (atrium/ventricles/both).

    endocardium
    both

11. Study Table 15.1 (p. 276 in *The Manual*) and reproduce it several times for your own benefit so you can anticipate when the doctor will call for transvenous pacemaker insertion.

The Pulse Generator *(pp. 276–279)*

We have an electrode in place to allow stimulation of the heart. Now we have to send an electrical current to the electrode. The device that sends the current is called a pacemaker or a pulse generator. It runs on batteries. This exercise reviews this magic little box.

Review 4

1. The simplest pacemaker uses a _____ or _____-rate pulse generator.

set-   fixed

2. If you set the pacing rate at 60, the generator fires _____ times per minute.

60

3. On the monitor you should see _____ pacemaker "blips" per minute. (See Figure 15–2 in *The Manual.*)

60

4. After each pacing blip you should see a wide _____.

QRS

5. This QRS resembles a _____ _____ _____ pattern.

bundle-branch block

6. If the heart beats by itself, the fixed-rate pacer (will/will not) fire anyway.

will

7. Thus, the pacemaker may _____ with the heart's natural impulses.

compete

8. As you remember, one of the dangers of PVCs is the _____ phenomenon, which can cause ventricular fibrillation.

R-on-T

9. Competition caused by pacing can also cause the _____ phenomenon if the pacing impulse strikes a T wave.

R-on-T

10. This, too, results in the potential threat of _____ _____.

ventricular fibrillation

"American ingenuity" came to the rescue, and the newer pacemakers use a *demand pulse generator*. How does this ingenious pacemaker operate?

Review 5

1. If a demand pacemaker senses a natural heartbeat, it (will/will not) fire.

will not

2. However, if the heart does not beat within a preset interval, the pacemaker will _____.

fire

3. When there is a natural, conducted heartbeat (R wave), the catheter tip transmits this information to a _____ device in the pacemaker.

sensing

4. When there is no natural heartbeat (no R wave), the pacemaker discharges an _____ _____ back to the heart.

electrical impulse

5. This type of pacemaker is called an R wave (inhibited/activated) pacemaker.

inhibited

6. The demand catheter has (1/2) function(s).

2

7. It serves as an ECG electrode to (send/sense) natural beats and as a pacing catheter to (send/sense) electrical stimuli.

sense
send

8. The demand pacemaker is designed to avoid _____ _____.

competition with the natural
   heartbeat

and therefore prevent _____ _____.

ventricular fibrillation

Catheter Electrodes *(pp. 279–280)*

Now that we have talked about different kinds of pacemakers, let's discuss different kinds of electrodes.

Review 6

1. To complete an electrical circuit, the pacemaker needs (1/2) electrode(s).

2

2. A unipolar catheter has (1/2) electrode(s) inside the heart, and one _____ the heart.

1   outside

3. The heart electrode is the (negative/positive) pole.

negative

4. The positive electrode is a wire suture in the _____.

skin

5. A bipolar catheter places (1/2) electrode(s) inside the heart.

2

6. Both electrodes are encased inside the _____.

catheter

7. (Bipolar/unipolar) pacing is most successful.

bipolar

Technique of Transvenous Pacing *(pp. 280–284)*

We are ready now to learn about inserting and using a pacemaker. We will stress the nursing role all the way through.

Review 7

1. The four veins generally used to insert a transvenous pacing electrode are _____, _____, _____, or _____.

femoral   jugular
antecubital   subclavian

2. Which veins are the most desirable? _____ or _____.

Jugular   subclavian

3. The catheter is threaded from the vein into the _____ _____, to the right _____, to the right _____.

vena cava
atrium   ventricle

4. Before the catheter is inserted, you will need supplies for _____ and _____ the skin.

cleaning
draping

5. Catheter insertion is usually performed through a large, special _____.

needle

6. Or a _____-_____ incision may be needed.

cut-down

7. Thus, you should have a _____-_____ tray handy.

cut-down

8. The electrode catheter is passed from the _____, _____, or _____ vein into the _____ _____ _____, into the _____ _____, through the _____ valve, and into the _____ _____.

antecubital   jugular
subclavian   superior vena cava
right atrium   tricuspid
right ventricle

9. The doctor may use _____ to see where the catheter is going.

fluoroscopy

10. In the CCU, the doctor can follow the catheter by means of an _____.

ECG

11. Then you (would/would not) attach four limb leads to the patient.

would

12. The free end of the catheter attaches to the _____ lead of the ECG with an alligator clip.

chest (or V)

13. The tracing is called an _____ ECG.

intracavitary

14. The pacemaker has _____ terminals for connecting the catheter.

two

15. These are marked _____ and _____.

negative   positive

16. With a unipolar catheter, insert the free end into the (negative/positive) terminal.

negative

17. The positive terminal would be connected to a _____ _____ _____.

wire skin suture

18. With a bipolar catheter, either wire can be connected to negative or positive terminals. (True/False)

True

When the catheter is in and attached to the pacemaker, how fast should the heart be paced?

19. The pacing rate must be (faster/slower) than the existing heart rate.

faster

20. If the pacing rate is too fast, the patient may complain of _____.

angina

21. Too fast rates may also (decrease/increase) ventricular filling and thus (decrease/increase) cardiac output.

decrease, decrease

22. Too slow rates might permit _____ arrhythmias to develop.

ectopic

In addition to the rate dial, your pacemaker will have an energy or intensity setting. How is this set?

23. The (lowest/highest) electrical setting that causes a contraction is the threshold level.	lowest
24. Settings lower than threshold (will/will not) cause contractions.	will not
25. Settings higher than threshold (will/will not) cause stronger contractions.	will not
26. To find the threshold level, start with the (lowest/highest) setting on the dial.	lowest
27. Increase the setting until you see a _____ with each pacing impulse.	QRS
28. This is the _____ level.	threshold
29. The usual level is less than _____ milliamperes.	two
30. The threshold level (does/does not) vary with time and electrode contact.	does
31. Thus the energy setting is usually set (higher/lower) than threshold.	higher
32. This energy setting is scaled in _____.	milliamperes
33. The pacemaker is usually left in the heart as long as _____ _____ _____ _____ _____ persist.	heart block or other arrhythmias
34. This is seldom over _____ days.	ten
35. But it may be left in a _____ longer, "just in case."	week

You can bet that your patient or his family will ask you, "Nurse, how long will this pacemaker be left in?" While the patient's doctor will decide, you should have some idea of what to expect.

Problems with Temporary Transvenous Pacing *(pp. 284–285)*

Pacemakers can save lives, but they can also cause some problems. As with any machine, all sorts of things can go wrong, and you need to know about these problems.

Review 8

1. To pace effectively, the electrode tip should touch the inner _____ of the ventricle.	wall (endocardium)
2. If it doesn't, pacing _____ may occur.	failure
3. This type of pacing failure is called _____ of _____.	loss capture
4. Loss of capture means that the pacemaker is firing but the heart isn't _____ in response to it.	beating
5. In this situation, the doctor may have to _____ the catheter.	reposition
6. In the meantime, you can try _____ _____.	changing the patient's position
7. For example, if the patient turned over in bed and capture is lost, try turning him _____.	back
8. Catheters inserted in the (arm/neck) are more prone to loss of capture.	arm
9. If the heart initiates its own beats between pacemaker-induced beats, we say _____ exists.	competition
10. Competition is more common with (fixed/demand) pacing.	fixed
11. However, a demand pacemaker may fire unnecessarily if the patient's QRS is too _____ to be sensed.	small
12. If you suddenly see no pacing blips on the monitor, the pacemaker (is/is not) functioning.	is not
13. Quickly, check the pacemaker to see if the pulse _____ (usually a flashing light) is working.	indicator

14. If the battery isn't firing, don't waste time. The problem then is with the battery, not the patient or electrode position. If this is the case, replace the _____.

| battery

15. Make sure all connections are _____.

| tight

16. Be ready to start _____ _____.

| cardiopulmonary resuscitation

17. If your patient's chest muscles begin to twitch during pacing, the electrodes may have _____ the ventricle wall.

| perforated

18. This may also cause contractions of the _____.

| diaphragm

19. Perforation usually (does/does not) cause dangerous bleeding from the ventricle.

| does not

20. If perforation occurs, the doctor will have to _____ the catheter.

| reposition

21. Infection of the catheter insertion site can be minimized by _____ _____ during insertion and the use of _____ _____ afterwards.

| aseptic
| technique   antibiotic ointment

22. After pacemaker insertion, watch the veins (especially in the arm) for signs of _____.

| thrombophlebitis or inflammation

Nursing Responsibility in Temporary Transvenous Cardiac Pacing (pp. 285–286)
Review 9

Dr. Hart says, "We are going to put in a pacemaker." What do you bring to the scene? Answer the following questions and then read the discussion that accompanies the answers. It will make this exercise more helpful if you can imagine yourself "flying" around collecting all these items while Dr. Hart impatiently taps his foot!

1. How do you prepare a conscious patient for an elective insertion? _____ _____

   How about during an emergency? _____ _____

2. What procedures do you follow to treat PVCs and ventricular fibrillation? _____ _____

3. "Monitoring" the catheter during insertion requires: _____ _____

4. Skin preparation requires: _____ _____

5. Draping requires: _____ _____

6. Catheter insertion requires: _____ _____

7. Catheter securing requires: _____ _____

8. While the doctor is busy inserting the catheter, who watches the ECG or monitor? ___ _____

Answers and Discussion

1. Preparing the patient for an elective insertion means *explaining*. Emphasize the positive and relate it to the familiar. You might say something like "You know, when you have an infection we can help your body by giving you a dose of penicillin or another antibiotic. Now, if your heart needs help, we can give it a 'dose' of pacemaker." You may frighten a patient who isn't comfortable with your terminology if you say "This is a prophylactic measure which we will activate if you go into complete heart block

to prevent your heart from going into ventricular fibrillation. It emits bursts of electricity that are conducted to your heart by . . ." Pretty scary stuff, right?

Most hospitals require a *"permit"* for elective procedures such as this. Know your hospital's policy.

In an emergency? *Try to save the patient's life first.* Someone should explain the procedure to the family, and some hospitals may obtain consent from family members to insert the pacemaker. If you are setting up for an emergency insertion, delegate the explanations and permission business to others.

2. PVCs and ventricular fibrillation during pacemaker insertion? Yes, they are both possible any time. Have a *patent IV* and *lidocaine* handy. Bring the *defibrillator* to the scene, plug it in, and screen it (if the patient is conscious) before the insertion is attempted.

3. For "monitoring" during an insertion you need an *ECG, limb leads,* and an *alligator clamp.* The ECG should be battery-operated; if not, be sure you ground it! Put the limb leads on the patient. After the catheter is inserted into the vein, connect the ECG chest lead to the catheter with an alligator clamp.

4. You will need *skin cleaning and antiseptic supplies.* You will have to find out what the doctor likes. Some want "that red stuff"; some like sprays; some swab it on. In an emergency, cleanse the skin with any antiseptic you have on hand, and don't worry.

5. *Drapes,* such as an "eye drape," small wound drape, or sterile towels, are needed. A sterile draw sheet, if you have one, turns the whole area into a "sterile" field.

6. *Cut-down set, local anesthetic, needle placement set*—don't forget the pacing catheters and the pacemaker! And just about now you will be sending for size 8 1/2 gloves instead of size 8. Once things get started, it's very handy if you can put on one sterile glove—then you can help in both the sterile field and with the unsterile pacemaker.

7. The catheter is in, you connect it, watch the monitor, and hooray! There's a QRS after every pacemaker blip. Now you will need to secure the catheter: *sutures, tape, antibiotic ointment, and dressings.*

8. You do!

MONITOR PRACTICE

Review 10

The pacemaker is in; the doctor goes home. Who must make sure "all systems are go"? You, right? Now, suppose that your patient's monitor suddenly looks like this:

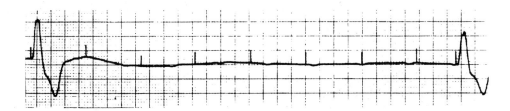

Figure 15.1

What do you do?

1. Check the patient's _____ and _____ _____.   pulse   blood pressure

2. _____ his position.   Change

3. _____ the doctor.   Notify

4. If necessary, start _____.   CPR

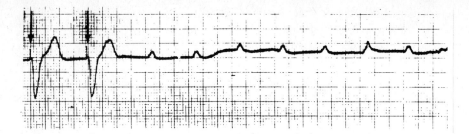

Figure 15.2

Review 11

Another patient's monitor shows this tracing (Fig. 15.2). What do you do?

1. First, make sure catheter terminals are not _____ or _____.   disconnected   loose

2. Check the _____ _____ on the pacemaker to see if the battery is firing.   pulse indicator

3. If not, _____ the battery. (You should have a standby battery.)   replace

4. Start _____ if necessary.   CPR

5. _____ the doctor.   Notify

6. If you notice competition, you _____ the doctor.   notify

7. If you notice twitching of the chest muscles, you _____ the doctor.   notify

8. Twice a day, at least, check the insertion site for _____ or _____.   infection   inflammation

See if you can interpret what the monitor tells you about pacemaker function. I have selected a series of monitor strips for us to analyze.

Review 12

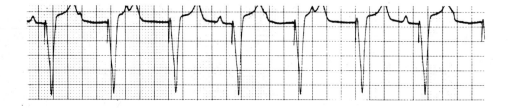

Figure 15.3. Patient 1.

This is a fixed-rate pacemaker.

1. Is it capturing? _____   Yes

2. Is there any competition? _____   No

3. Is the pacemaker functioning well? _____   Yes

4. What is the pacing rate? _____   About 70 beats/min

5. Are there any P waves? _____   Yes

6. Do they have any relationship to the QRS complexes? _____   No

7. What type of heart block do you think the pacemaker is being used for? _____ _____   Third degree

Review 13

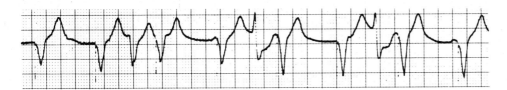

Figure 15.4. Patient 2.

1. Is it a fixed-rate or a demand pacemaker? _____   Fixed-rate

2. Are there any natural heartbeats seen? _____   Yes

3. Does the pacemaker recognize them? _____   No

4. What is the danger of this? _____.   The pacing impulse may strike a T wave

5. This could result in _____ _____.   ventricular fibrillation

6. What should you do? _____.   Tell the doctor

Review 14

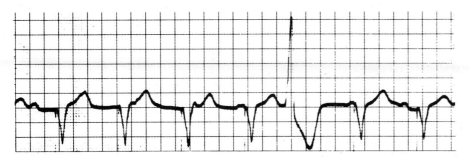

Figure 15.5. Patient 3.

1. What kind of pacemaker is this? _____   Demand

2. Is it functioning well? _____   Yes

3. What did the pacemaker do when it recognized a PVC? _____   It didn't fire, and reset itself

   _____.

Review 15

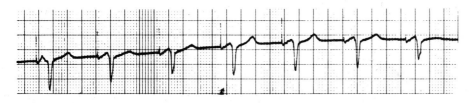

Figure 15.6. Patient 4.

1. Are the pacing spikes regular? _____   Yes

2. Do the QRS complexes show the customary bundle-branch pattern? _____   No

3. Why not? _____   The pacemaker is in the atrium; this is atrial pacing

   _____.

Review 16

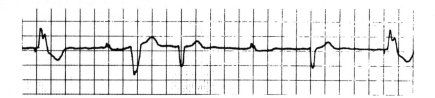

Figure 15.7. Patient 5.

1. The first and last beats on this strip show that pacemaker stimulus _____ the ventricles.

    captures

2. But in between these two beats, the pacing stimulus produces no _____.

    response

3. There has been loss of _____ during this period.

    capture

4. Is this dangerous? _____

    Yes

5. What should you do? _____.

    Notify the doctor

6. What is the most likely cause of this problem? _____ _____.

    Displacement of the catheter tip

7. What will have to be done? _____ _____.

    Probably reposition the catheter

PERMANENT CARDIAC PACING *(pp. 287–289)*

Who needs a permanent cardiac pacemaker? Table 15.3 (p. 287, *The Manual*) spells it out in detail. But before we get too complex, grab hold of two words: bradycardia and symptomatic. Makes sense, doesn't it? If the heart rate is so inadequate that the patient has symptoms he can't live with, something has to be done. So let's put long-suffering Mr. Kardiak into complete heart block and discuss permanent pacing.

Review 17

1. Look at Table 15.3 (p. 287, *The Manual*), Class I, Section A. Summing it up, if Mr. Kardiak has _____, a pacemaker is indicated.

    symptoms

2. His symptoms might include _____, _____, _____, _____ _____ etc.

    CHF ectopics confusion unconsciousness

3. Now suppose Mr. Kardiak has second-degree heart block with a ventricular rate below _____ and has symptoms, is a permanent pacemaker indicated? _____

    40 Yes

4. Take a look at the monitor next door to Mr. Kardiak. The monitor shows first-degree AV block (ie, P–R longer than _____) does this patient need a permanent pacemaker? _____

    0.20 sec
    No

5. In between these two extremes is the gray area where doctors don't agree on the need for permanent pacemakers. Again the key word in determining is if the patient is _____.

    symptomatic

6. A class I or II with (asymptomatic/symptomatic) patient is in the gray area.

    asymptomatic

7. A complete heart block with heart rate (above/below) 40 is in the gray area also.

    above

Types of Permanent Cardiac Pacemakers *(pp. 287–289)*
Review 18

1. Back to basics—the first permanent pacemaker was one electrode in the _____ _____ and pace 'em!

    right ventricle

2. Then it was realized that the "atrial kick" increased the ventricular output _____ to _____%.

    20
    30

3. So now we have permanent pacemakers that preserve _____ _____.

    AV synchrony

4. This means that the _____ systole precedes the _____ systole in an appropriate timing.

    atrial   ventricular

5. The atria need to be synchronized to contract (prior to/after) the ventricular contraction.

    prior to

6. This allows the _____ to empty more completely and to _____ ventricular output 20 to 30%.

    atria   increase

7. This also (increases/decreases) atrial pressure and allows increased _____ return to the atria.

    decreases   venous

8. The old pacemakers were _____ rate. If the patient's rate was set at 70 and he ran a marathon, his heart rate stayed at _____.

    fixed
    70

9. Now permanent pacemakers are _____ responsive; this is especially good for _____ people.

    rate
    younger

10. Now permanent pacemakers can be AV _____, _____-modulated and, add to that, _____.

    synchronized   rate
    multiprogrammable

11. Look at Table 15.4 (p. 288, *The Manual*). In a pacemaker code, the first letter refers to the chamber _____, the second letter to the chamber _____, and the third letter refers to the _____ _____ _____.

    paced   sensed
    mode of response

12. If there are five letters on a pacemaker code, the fourth letter refers to the _____ functions.

    programmable

13. The fifth letter refers to the (tachyarrhythmia/bradyarrhythmia) function.

    tachyarrhythmia

14. Now look at Table 15.5 (p. 288, *The Manual*). Without using Table 14.4, figure out the pacemaker codes. The first one is AAI. The first A, the chamber paced, is the _____. The second A in the code, the chamber sensed, is the _____. And the I refers to the _____ _____ _____ and shows it is _____ when an electrical impulse from the _____ is sensed. Do the rest of them and check yourself on Table 15.4 (p. 288, *The Manual*).

    atrium   atrium
    mode of response
    inhibited   heart

15. In symptomatic bradycardia the pacemaker of choice is _____ because it paces and senses in the _____.

    VVI
    ventricles

16. If there is an AV block, the pacemaker indicated is a VDD because it is _____ triggered and _____ inhibited.

    atrially   ventricularly

Procedure of Permanent Pacemaker Implantation *(p. 289)*
Review 19

Let's prepare Mr. Kardiak and his family for a permanent pacemaker implantation. After you have carefully explained the reason for the pacemaker:

1. Mr. Kardiak asks: How big is it? What does it look like? Your best answer: _____
_____

    Show him the real thing or at least a picture.

2. Mrs. Kardiak asks: Will he be asleep? _____
_____

    No, but he will be kept comfortable.

3. Mr. Kardiak says: You'll do it right here in CCU, won't you? _____
_____
_____

No, they need fluoroscopy and a sterile environment.

4. Mrs. Kardiak says: The doctor says they insert the leads like an IV. But where? _____
_____
_____

Show them, the subclavian or jugular veins.

5. Mr. Kardiak is looking worriedly at the pulse generator. Where does that go? _____
_____
_____

Show him, under the skin below the clavicle.

6. Mrs. Kardiak asks: How long will he have to stay in bed after? _____
_____
_____

24 hours

7. Mr. Kardiak asks: Didn't the doctor say something about antibiotics? _____
_____
_____

Yes, for 24 hours

16

Treatment of Life-threatening Arrhythmias: Implantable Defibrillators, Radiofrequency Ablation, and Precordial Shock

Electrophysiologic Studies *(p. 291)*
Review 1

1. If just plain monitoring and a 12-lead ECG do not identify arrhythmias, a 24-hour monitor (ie, _____ monitor) can be used or monitoring during exercise (ie, _____ testing) may be tried.

   Holter
   stress

2. If these are inadequate, EPS (spell it out once, please) _____ _____ can be performed.

   electrophysiologic studies

3. The EPS procedure is similar to cardiac _____.

   catheterization

4. Special catheters are placed in the _____ side of the heart.

   right

5. Electrical recordings can be made of the _____ pathways and the mechanisms of _____ can be identified.

   conduction
   arrhythmias

6. Pacing _____ can be delivered at specific _____ in the cardiac cycle.

   stimuli   intervals

7. This is called _____ _____ stimulation.

   programmed electrical

8. An "inducible" arrhythmia" must be (1) induced by _____ _____, (2) sustained longer than _____ seconds, and (3) cause altered _____.

   electrical
     stimulation   30
   hemodynamics

9. Inducible arrhythmias are related to _____ mechanisms.

   re-entry

10. Non-inducible arrhythmias are usually related to enhanced _____.

    automaticity .

197

Review 2

I remember a sweet little lady, the wife of a retired pediatrician. She kept going into ventricular fibrillation for no reason that could be identified. The first time it happened, she was in CCU. The second time, she was in ER. Her husband bought a portable defibrillator and learned how to use it. He defibrillated her several times—at home, in the car, and places they visited. And then one day he wasn't right at her elbow and she died. Oh, how I wish we had had AICDs before 1985.

1. AICD: spell it out once, please: _____ _____ _____ _____ _____.

> automatic implantable cardioverter defibrillator

2. Patients treated with AICDs have an annual mortality rate of less than _____%.

> 5

3. Patients without AICDs, treated with medications, have a mortality rate of about _____%.

> 40

4. One class of patients who are appropriate for AICD are those who have survived a cardiac _____ not associated with an _____.

> arrest   AMI

5. The other class are those who in the EPS lab using _____ _____ stimulation go into _____ arrhythmias (eg, sustained hypotensive _____ _____ or _____ _____).

> programmed electrical inducible ventricular tachycardia ventricular fibrillation

6. If you have never seen an AICD, look at Figure 16–1 (p. 292, *The Manual*). The parts are: a _____ implanted in an _____ _____ pocket and _____ or _____ leads for rate sensing and defibrillation.

> generator   abdominal wall transvenous   epicardial

7. In general, AICDs monitor _____ activity and _____ tachyarrhythmias with cardioversion or _____.

> cardiac   treat defibrillation

8. Most AICDs sense the heart _____ and the _____ of the ECG tracing.

> rate   shape

9. Most AICDs are programmed to measure the length of time the ECG complex remains on the _____ line.

> isoelectric

10. This is called the _____ _____ _____ or PDF.

> probability density function

11. If the complex remains off the isoelectric line more than _____% of the time or the _____ exceeds the limits, the AICD will defibrillate.

> 50
> rate

12. Do newer units use both criteria? _____

> Yes

13. The AICD can deliver _____ or _____ shocks.

> 4   5

14. Newer AICDs can do (1) _____ or defibrillation, (2) overdrive pacing for _____ pacing, (3) ventricular demand pacing for _____. (Next, we will have a choice of jazz or waltz rhythm!)

> cardioversion antitachycardic bradycardias

Patient Preparation *(p. 292)*

Review 3

Put yourself in this patient's place. Can't you imagine yourself thinking: "What if this hauls off and kicks me when I don't need it? Or worse, what if it doesn't work when I do need it? This will be like living with a time bomb inside of me." The patient and family need every bit of information you can give them: booklets, pamphlets, video tapes. A scrapbook of successful patients would be wonderful!

1. In addition to information about AICDs, this patient needs basic general surgical preparation, eg, _____ breathing and _____.

deep   coughing

2. Insertion of AICD may be through a _____ incision or _____. (You and the patient need to know which.)

thoracotomy   transvenous

3. With a thoracotomy the patient may have _____ tubes for a day or two.

chest

4. Then you will be concerned with preventing pulmonary complications with _____ _____, _____, and incentive _____.

deep breathing
coughing   spirometry

5. You need to know exactly which _____ of AICD was implanted and what to expect and what to do if something goes wrong!

type

6. Before the patient goes home he must have the following information: (1) AICD's model _____ and _____, (2) _____ number for follow-up care, (3) _____ rate detection level, and (4) _____ cut-off rate.

name   number   telephone
tachycardia   bradycardia

7. The patient should be given a list (provided by the manufacturer of the AICD) of electromagnetic interference sources, eg, large _____ speakers, _____ wands, industrial _____, and _____ machines.

stereo   bingo
transformers   MRI

RADIOFREQUENCY ABLATION (pp. 293–294)

Review 4

1. Radiofrequency ablation is usually done when an _____ study is done.

EPS

2. It is used to treat _____ and _____ problems that are unresponsive to drug treatment.

arrhythmias   conduction

3. The patient (will/will not) be anesthetized and (will/will not) be sedated.

will not   will

4. Drugs suggested for sedation are _____ and _____.

midazolam   meperidine

5. Drugs that might be used for diagnostic purposes include _____ and _____.

isoproterenol
adenosine

6. Usually, four _____ are inserted under fluoroscopy.

catheters

7. Three catheters are introduced through the _____ vein into the right _____, _____ _____ area and the right _____.

femoral
atrium   His bundle   ventricle

8. The fourth catheter is inserted through the internal _____ or _____ vein.

jugular   subclavian

9. This is then introduced into the _____ _____.

coronary sinus

10. If the left side of the heart must be reached, that catheter goes in through the _____ artery.

femoral

11. Each catheter has multiple electrodes to help identify the _____ of the arrhythmias (called endocardial _____).

site
mapping

12. Once a site is identified, _____ is sent through the catheter to "cauterize" the tissue.

current

13. The current delivered to the endocardium is _____-voltage, _____-frequency alternating current. Does the patient feel this? _____

low   high
No

14. If an inducible arrhythmia persists, current can be delivered again to cauterize or to create another "_____."

lesion

15. The lesions created are only several _____.

millimeters

16. The objective is to cauterize the areas responsible for _____ rhythms or that are _____ _____ for ventricular tachycardia.

re-entry
ectopic foci

17. One indication for ablation is AV nodal _____ tachycardia. | re-entrant

18. Remember, in this arrhythmia there is a _____ and a _____ conduction pathway. (Go back to page 187 in *The Manual*.) | slow   fast

19. Experience shows that it is better to cauterize the (slow/fast) pathway. | slow

20. Cauterizing the (slow/fast) pathway can cause complete heart block. | fast

21. The ablation procedure usually lasts _____ to _____ hours but can last as long as _____ hours. | 2   4
10

22. Ablation is about (65/75/95)% successful. | 95

23. Post-op care is similar to that of a patient who has had coronary _____ or catheterization. | angiography

24. Patients will receive _____ if they have had arterial cannulation. | heparin

25. Patients are discharged on low-dose _____ or _____ for one month. | warfarin   aspirin

PRECORDIAL SHOCK *(pp. 294–299)*

Review 5

1. One form of electric shock is called defibrillation. (True/False) | True

2. Defibrillation is used to terminate _____ _____. | ventricular fibrillation

3. Defibrillation is an emergency life-saving measure. (True/False) | True

4. Defibrillation uses a _____ voltage shock. | high

5. It stops (all/some) of the heart's electrical activity for a fraction of a second. | all

6. Then, hopefully, normal sinus rhythm re-establishes itself. (True/False) | True

7. The chances for successful defibrillation (increase/decrease) with any delay in performing the procedure. | decrease

8. Defibrillation is a term also used for elective treatment of arrhythmias. (True/False) | False

9. The second form of precordial shock is called _____. | cardioversion

10. Cardioversion can be used to terminate _____ as well as ventricular arrhythmias. | atrial

11. Cardioversion is an elective, therapeutic measure. (True/False) | True

12. The basic electrical principles of cardioversion and defibrillation (are/are not) the same. | are

13. However, _____ must be used at a particular time in the cardiac cycle. | cardioversion

14. _____ is not synchronized with any part of the cardiac cycle. | Defibrillation

15. Both types of shock can be delivered by the same machine. (True/False) | True

Equipment for Precordial Shock *(p. 295)*
Review 6

1. You are most likely to find (AC/DC) defibrillators in your hospital. | DC

2. DC defibrillators can be used for (both/one) kind(s) of shock. | both

3. When you turn the defibrillator on, it first (stores/delivers) electrical energy. | stores

4. When you press the discharge switch, it (stores/delivers) electrical energy. | delivers

5. The amount of electrical current actually delivered to the heart is affected by transthoracic _____.

impedance

6. Impedance is the _____ to current flow.

resistance

7. Impedance is measured in _____.

ohms

8. Impedance is affected by the _____ of the paddles and how they are applied.

size

9. You need to use a conductive _____ or _____-_____ pads to improve conduction.

cream (jel) saline-soaked

10. You apply the paddles (very lightly/very firmly) to the chest.

very firmly

11. The chest size (ie, the distance to the _____) can affect conduction.

heart

12. Repeated shocks and the time interval between each (do/do not) affect conduction.

do

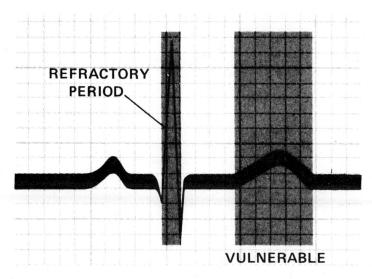

Figure 16.1

Synchronized and Nonsynchronized Precordial Shock *(p. 295)*

Before we begin the next section, do you remember the R-on-T phenomenon? If not, study Figure 16.1 (above) and answer the following.

Review 7

1. An R-on-T type PVC can theoretically cause _____ _____.

ventricular fibrillation

2. Precordial shock striking on the T wave (could/could not) possibly cause ventricular fibrillation.

could

3. In treating atrial arrhythmias with shock, you (could/could not) possibly hit the T.

could

4. So you could possibly convert atrial arrhythmias to ventricular _____.

fibrillation

5. Would you ever want to do this? _____

NO, NO, NO!

6. The T wave is in the (vulnerable/nonvulnerable) period in the cardiac cycle.

vulnerable

7. The nonvulnerable period is also called the _____ period.

refractory

8. The QRS is in the (vulnerable/refractory) period.

refractory

9. Synchronized shock is delivered in the (vulnerable/refractory) period.

refractory

10. The defibrillator does this by recognizing the _____ complex and firing at that time.

QRS

11. The synchronizer switch must be (on/off) for a defibrillator to sense the QRS wave. — on

12. In ventricular fibrillation, _____ complexes do not exist. — QRS

13. Thus, if the synchronizer is on, the machine (can/cannot) find an R wave to discharge on. — cannot

14. If you have the synchronizer on, can you treat ventricular fibrillation? _____ — No

15. If you have the synchronizer on, can you treat atrial fibrillation? _____ — Yes

16. If you have the synchronizer *off*, can you treat ventricular fibrillation? _____ — Yes

17. If you have the synchronizer *off*, can you safely treat atrial fibrillation? _____ — No

18. Do you fully understand questions 14–17? _____
(If not, reread this section in *The Manual*.)

Dr. Hart calls and says, "I'll be in within 15 minutes to use synchronized shock on the patient with atrial fibrillation." What do you do?

Review 8

1. First, _____ the procedure to the patient. — explain

2. Have the patient sign a _____. — permit or release

3. Bring the _____ to the bedside. — machine

(If your defibrillator has a built-in synchronizer, that's only one piece of equipment you will need. If not, you will need a defibrillator and a synchronizer, plus the cords to connect them.)

4. Emergency supplies you may need should be on your _____ _____. Bring it to the bedside. — crash cart

5. Supplies should include a syringe containing 100-mg _____. — lidocaine

6. Resuscitation equipment should include: _____, _____ _____, _____ _____. — airways   breathing bag   cardiac board

7. You should have an _____ line in place in this patient. — IV

8. Some type of _____ or sedation will be needed for the shock. — anesthetic

9. _____ the patient that sedation will make the procedure quite tolerable. — Reassure

If you bring this equipment, one piece at a time, and prepare and assemble it in the patient's room, you are going to scare him so badly that you may never need the synchronizer! Reduce the fuss and apprehension to a minimum.

Review 9

If your synchronizer is separate from your defibrillator, be sure not only to read the instructions for this machine, but to practice assembling the pieces. The doctors will expect you to set up the equipment; in fact, they may not be familiar with your hospital's synchronizer at all. These general concepts should apply to almost any kind of synchronizer.

1. You first turn the synchronizer switch _____. — on

2. The synchronizer needs an _____ wave to synchronize itself on. — R or QRS

3. If the patient's QRS is too _____, the synchronizer may not recognize it. — small or low

4. Adjust the gain dial to get sufficient _____ of the QRS. — height or voltage

5. Some synchronizers can be set to recognize (negative/positive/both) R waves. _____ How about yours? _____ — Both

6. The doctor determines the _____ setting.

watt-second

7. Some type of short-acting _____ is usually used for elective shock. Be sure to find out what drugs you will need for this.

anesthetic

Automated External Defibrillators *(pp. 295–296)*
Review 8

For just a second, step out of CCU and ride in the ambulance bringing in your next patient.

1. _____ _____ defibrillators are used by ACLS (_____ _____ _____ _____) providers.

Automated external
Advanced Cardiac Life
  Support

2. Two _____ _____ (electrodes) are applied to the patient in place of defibrillator paddles.

adhesive pads

3. In the _____ mode, if the defibrillator recognizes _____ _____ it will deliver a shock.

automatic   ventricular
  fibrillation

4. In the semi-automatic or shock-advisory mode, what does it do? _____ _____

Sends message to shock.

5. The operator (can/cannot) override the machine.

can

Energy of Discharge *(p. 296)*
Review 9

1. Back in CCU, it is recommended that for the first defibrillation attempt you set the energy level at _____ J.

200

2. If needed, you give the second shock at _____ to _____ J.

200   300

3. For a third shock, increase the energy level to _____ J.

360

4. After three unsuccessful shocks, it's time to start assisted _____ and give _____ _____ mg IV.

ventilation
Epinephrine 1

5. And then _____.

repeat the shocks

6. Shocks greater than _____ J are not indicated for very large patients.

360

7. Switch mental gears to cardioversion: energy setting then (does/does not) vary with the type of arrhythmia.

does

8. Atrial flutter and SPVT can usually be terminated with _____ J.

50

9. Atrial fibrillation requires (50/100/150) J for successful treatment.

100

10. The morphology (form and structure) of ventricular tachycardia (does/does not) affect cardioversion.

does

11. Ventricular tachycardia that is regular in form and rate requires _____ J to convert.

100

12. In ventricular tachycardia that is irregular in rate and rhythm, you should start with a _____ J setting for cardioversion.

200

Technique of Elective Cardioversion and the Nursing Role *(pp. 296–298)*
Review 10

1. You first turn the synchronizer switch _____.

on

2. The synchronizer needs an _____ wave to synchronize itself on.

R or QRS

3. _____ levels should be drawn if the patient is on that drug.

Digitalis

4. Patients can be safely cardioverted with digoxin levels of _____ to _____ mg/mL. | 0.8 2.0

5. Adjust the gain dial to get sufficient _____ of the QRS. | height or voltage

6. Some synchronizers can be set to recognize (negative/positive/both) R waves. How about yours? _____ | both

7. The doctor determines the _____ setting. | watt-second

8. Some type of short-acting _____ is usually used for elective shock. Be sure to find out what drugs you will need for this. | anesthetic

9. Apply just the right amount of _____ _____ or _____ _____ to help prevent burns. | conductive jelly   electrode paste

10. Paste squishing out from beneath the paddles (can/cannot) cause sparks. | can

11. You will also need a _____ _____ and a _____ _____ cuff. | pulse oximeter   blood pressure

Technique of Emergency Defibrillation (p. 298)
Review 11

1. Ventricular fibrillation must be treated with _____. | defibrillation

2. Defibrillation should be done within _____ to _____ minutes after the onset of fibrillation. | 1   2

3. This means you _____ to the bedside if ventricular fibrillation occurs. | run, not walk

4. You (do/do not) have to wait for a doctor's order to defibrillate. (Unless your hospital policy says you must, which would be a shame.) | do not

5. Remember the energy settings? First shock, _____ J; second shock, _____ to _____ J; third shock, _____ J. | 200   200 300   360

6. And the synchronizer must be turned _____. | off

7. Do you check the monitor between shocks for a "normal" rhythm? _____ | Yes

8. If you continue to see ventricular fibrillation do you pause between shocks for anything else? _____ | No

9. Might you have to push a "recharge" button between shocks? _____ _____ | Maybe, know your equipment.

Review 12

Place an S in front of the terms that pertain to synchronized shock. Place a D in front of those that apply to defibrillation.

1. _____ elective | 1. S
2. _____ higher energy | 2. D
3. _____ nonsynchronized | 3. D
4. _____ cardioversion | 4. S
5. _____ anesthesia | 5. S
6. _____ two minutes | 6. D
7. _____ ventricular fibrillation | 7. D
8. _____ permit required | 8. S
9. _____ minimum energy | 9. S
10. _____ emergency | 10. D

Postresuscitation Care *(pp. 298–299)*
Review 13

In ordinary language, this patient will tell friends: "I died!" The emotional trauma and fear must be unimaginable. And yes, there may be sore muscles from the intense muscle contractions caused by the shock. And if there has been CPR—OUCH!

1. Of prime importance is _____ of a recurrence of the precipitating arrhythmia.

   prevention

2. Optimal tissue perfusion, especially to the _____ is another prime concern.

   brain

3. The patient must be carefully evaluated for (cardiovascular/pulmonary/neurological/ all three) conditions.

   all three

4. If the patient is comatose, you will need to insert a _____ catheter and if there are no bowel sounds, a _____ tube.

   urinary
   nasogastric

5. If the patient has had CPR he may have _____ _____ or at least, a very sore _____.

   rib fractures
   sternum

6. More serious, you watch for signs of pericardial _____ or _____ _____.

   tamponade
   hemopneumothorax

7. Remember the importance of YOUR reassurance and _____ to this patient.

   listening

You have finished the Reviews in this book. Be sure to study the appendixes in *The Manual,* pages 309–343, for more material that will help you. You are on your way now and here's hoping you will be the very best CCU nurse ever. And someday soon, let's see you at the desk, teaching a new CCU nurse.